SEASON OF SHADOWS
A FATHER'S GRIEF

By

Tom Hooker

God Bless

Tom Hooker

ISBN: 1-4033-0233-2 (ebook)
ISBN: 1-4033-0234-0 (softcover)

This book is printed on acid free paper.

1stBooks – rev. 3/22/02

For Elaine, my wife,
who dried my tears and salved my anger.

ALSO BY TOM HOOKER:

CALVARY'S CHILD:
THE LIFE OF AMANDA CAROL HOOKER

INTRODUCTION

"One day, a man was walking down a road, and he fell into a deep, dark hole. It was so deep and so dark, he couldn't get out. A short while later, a philanthropist came walking down the same road. This philanthropist was very rich, and had given millions of dollars to help the poor and needy.

"'Please, sir,' called the man. 'I've fallen into this hole, and I can't get out. Will you help me?'

"So the philanthropist wrote the man a large check and dropped it into the hole, and walked on. Some time later, a priest came walking down the road.

"'Please, sir,' called the man. 'I've fallen into this hole, and I can't get out. Will you help me?'

"So the priest wrote a prayer on a piece of paper, dropped it into the hole, and walked on. Not long after that, a friend came walking down the road.

"'Please, sir,' called the man. 'I've fallen into this hole, and I can't get out. Will you help me?'

"So the friend jumped down into the hole with the man.

"'Why did you do that?' asked the man. "Now both of us are stuck in the bottom of this hole!'

"'Yeah,' said the friend. 'But I've been here before, and I know the way out.'"

Leo McGarity to Josh Lyman in a scene from the NBC TV show *The West Wing.*

On December 1, 1997 I began my descent into the depths of clinical depression. By then, I had endured the

vii

first five months of what was to be the worst two years of my life. On that day, I glimpsed what the next eighteen months held in store.

In July 1997 my twenty-one year-old daughter began experiencing extreme nausea, and was unable to keep any food down. By the end of August, her stomach had stopped working completely. On September 12, her doctors found the cause. A cancerous tumor had sealed off the upper portion of her small intestine. Through Thanksgiving, her doctors efforts to restore her digestive function and to arrest the growth of the inoperative tumor had failed. Carol's oncologist arranged for her to see one of the world's best gastro-enterology oncologists at M. D. Anderson Cancer Clinic in Houston Texas. That doctor gave us a subtle message that Carol's condition was terminal.

Amanda Carol Hooker's death on February 10, 1998 ended a brief life spent in praise of God. She touched lives all over the world, and shared her love of Jesus with all she met. The story of Carol's life, her witness, and her struggle with cancer is recounted in the book *Calvary's Child: The Life of Amanda Carol Hooker.*

In this book, I hope to share my experiences during the sixteen-month period from December 1997 to March 1999. By sharing this journey I hope to provide encouragement to others who have made or who are making similar journeys, and to deliver the message, "You are not alone." I've been here before, and I know the way out.

By describing my emotions, I hope to help others understand that their emotions are not unique. I hope to enable others to realize that shock, despair, frustration and anger are part of the process of grieving – even for a Christian. God made us that way, and God understands how we feel.

By recounting my experiences with clinical depression, I hope to allay the fears of stigma that many sufferers have.

By describing the symptoms of the disease – which is a medical condition and not a mental illness – I hope to help those who unknowingly suffer from this disease identify their condition and seek professional help. By explaining the treatment I received and the improvement that treatment provided, I hope to encourage others to get help.

Within the pages of this book, I hope also to provide assurance to those who are making this journey that life will get better. I will never "recover" from the death of my daughter. I don't want to. But the burden of grief that once was so great is lighter now. I have the assurance that Carol is in Heaven. I find comfort in that. I am a different person than I was at the beginning of 1997. I have been changed forever, but I live on.

Most importantly, I want to use this book to emphasize that during all these months, Jesus never left my side. While I don't understand why my family had to endure this tragedy, I am convinced there is a way to praise God in it. I also believe that one day, In Heaven, I will understand and will agree with God's wisdom in this matter.

I am convinced that hardships such as this – and everyone endures a hardship of one kind or another – serve to forge a stronger bond between us and God if we will only allow it. Dietrich Bonhoeffer was a Christian minister who stood up for God in the face of Nazi oppression in 1930's and 1940's Germany. He was imprisoned in a Nazi concentration camp for two years before being executed in April 1945, only one month before Germany surrendered. In 1943, Bonhoeffer wrote these words to his sister, "It is good to learn early enough that suffering and God are not a contradiction but rather a unity, for the idea that God himself is suffering is one that has always been one of the most convincing teachings of Christianity. I think God is nearer to suffering than to happiness, and to find God in this way gives peace and rest and a strong and courageous heart."

When Bonhoeffer was hung in 1945, the Nazi doctor whose job was to observe the execution and certify his death recorded these words, "At the place of execution, he again said a short prayer and then climbed the steps to the gallows, brave and composed...In the almost fifty years that I worked as a doctor, I have hardly ever seen a man die so entirely submissive to the will of God."

Only by enduring the pain of this life are we able to comprehend the depth of the pain that Jesus experienced – for us – on the cross. Only by enduring the pain of this life are we able to anticipate the joy that awaits us in Heaven.

There is one last thing that I hope to convey in this book. I offer a reminder that hardships such as these equip us to serve God *now*. By enduring the trials of this life we are better able to see and understand the trials of others who face similar hardships. Philo of Alexandria said, "Be kind, for everyone you meet is fighting a great battle." Everyone endures suffering, and they need our help and God's to do it. The Army drill sergeant who guides the recruit through strenuous basic training has been through basic training himself.

I pray, then, that this book will be a handkerchief which dries the tears of those who suffer, a beacon which lights the way for those who stumble along a dangerous and unfamiliar path, and a door which leads to a new resolve to praise and serve God.

CHAPTER ONE

"Then one of the synagogue rulers, named Jairus, came there. Seeing Jesus, he fell at His feet and pleaded earnestly with him. 'My little daughter is dying. Please come and put your hands on her so that she will be healed and live.'" Mark 5:22-23

Two months. Sixty-nine days, in fact. That's how long we had from our return from the M.D. Anderson cancer clinic until Carol died. Such a short time.

In her book *After the Death of a Child*, Ann K. Finkbeiner reports that a characteristic of a parent who has lost a child is an increased sensitivity to others' pain. In my lifetime, I have read the Bible passage above dozens of thanks. Perhaps I thought about Jairus' desperation, but only in an offhand way. It wasn't until Carol became ill that I *really* understood how Jairus felt. I was there, in his shoes, at Jesus' feet, pleading for my child as well.

From the time of my birth until Carol became ill, I had never really experienced a crisis. Sure, my grandparents had died, and I had to deal with that. But part of life is burying your elder relatives, and that was something I could deal with. After I graduated from college, I only spent two months without a job. Early in our marriage, we struggled with a tight budget, but once again, that is nothing unusual. For the past twenty years we were financially stable – not wealthy – but we paid the bills. Perhaps I had gotten smug, thinking that I had surmounted all of life's obstacles, and that my life was going to be "smooth sailing". Carol's illness changed all that very quickly.

I was born in Pontotoc, Mississippi and grew up in rural farm country in nearby Thaxton. When I give my testimony, I ask my listeners if they are familiar with the reference to a person who is "born with a silver spoon in his mouth." Of course, that refers to a person born into a wealthy household, who has no concerns for his physical needs. I was not born with a silver spoon in my mouth. My family was poor, but no poorer than my neighbors. In that time and place, there just wasn't much money floating around. We always had food on the table, however, and clean clothes. I may have had a patch on the knee of my jeans, but that isn't unusual for an active boy. I was fortunate to be born into a household that was rich in love. My childhood home was filled with a love for Jesus, and a love for each other. That kind of wealth is greater than the other kind, anyway.

While I wasn't born with a silver spoon in my mouth, I was born with a hammer in my hand. I don't remember when I first used that hammer. I probably disobeyed one of my parents, when I knew better. Or I may have told a "little white lie", or I may have stolen a nickel or a pencil from a schoolmate. When I did that. I swung the hammer, and began to drive nails into the hands and feet of Jesus.

I have heard the testimonies of such men as Mike Warnke, who was a high priest of a satanic coven in California, and Don Babbin and Freddie Gage, who at different times led criminal gangs in Houston, Texas. They tell stories of the terrible sins they committed, and how Jesus forgave them of those sins when they repented and asked for salvation. I haven't done any such "terrible" things, but the sins that I did commit condemned me to Hell just as surely as murder would have. I was just another sinner hammering away at those nails.

I mentioned earlier that I was raised in a household that loved Jesus. Both my parents were strong Christians. I spent many hours inside Thaxton Baptist Church. I attended Sunday School and worship on Sunday morning, and Training Union and worship on Sunday night. I went to prayer meeting on Wednesday night. I was a member of the Royal Ambassadors (kind of like Boy Scouts with a missions emphasis), and I attended Vacation Bible School every summer. I was well educated in the tenets of Christianity. This served to prepare me for the day when I encountered Jesus.

In those days mechanical cotton pickers were not in common use. Most of the people in Thaxton who farmed harvested their cotton crops by hand. This usually began in September and continued through October. Since those of us who attended school were needed as field hands, we began our school year in the middle of July and attended school for six weeks. Then school dismissed for six weeks so the cotton crop could be "brought in." Believe me, there are few things less fun than attending school in an un-air conditioned Mississippi schoolhouse in July!

Thus, I was in school during the first week of August, 1959. That same week, Thaxton Baptist Church held its summer revival. In those days, revival week meant two services a day. The first was held at 10:00 in the morning, and the second was held at 7:00 at night. Most of the women in the community were housewives, and they were the primary attendees at the morning service. The men attended if the weather was too bad to tend the fields. Also, the principal pulled a bus up to the front door of the school, and any student who wanted to attend the revival was excused from class long enough to attend. My, how times have changed!

I chose to attend the revival. For one thing, it would get me out of the classroom for an hour, although I'm not sure why a seven-year old boy would find sitting in a church sanctuary preferable to sitting in a classroom. For another thing, attending revival would get me some brownie points from Mom, which always came in handy when I found myself in a tight spot.

3

So, when Brother Billy Baker, our evangelist for the week, stood for his message that Friday morning, I was in the congregation. Somewhere during the service, Brother Baker sang a song made famous by Tennessee Ernie Ford, "Wayfaring Stranger." I know this is pretty heavy thinking for a seven-year old, but I realized I was indeed a wayfaring stranger. This wasn't my home. I was destined for another home "over Jordan". I realized that I couldn't get there by myself. I was lost. I had sinned, and that sin separated me from Jesus. When the invitation was given, I responded. I don't remember this, but Mother tells me I jumped over two church pews to get to the altar. Brother Robert Deline, Thaxton's pastor, took me into one of the Sunday School classrooms and talked with me about salvation.

With his help, and using the information I had learned during my years in church, I realized the only way I could reach my home over Jordan was to put my faith in Jesus. I asked Jesus to forgive me, and to save me. In that moment, I symbolically raised the hand that held the hammer I had carried since birth. Jesus took that hammer from my hand, and placed His hand in mine. Since that day, I have walked hand in hand with Jesus.

I wish I could say that since that day, I have lived a sin-free life. I can't. Unfortunately, my human weakness has caused me to do things that Jesus doesn't want me to do, and to fail to do something that He does want. I can say, however, that I have lived a forgiven life, and that is even better. One of the things that this forgiven life provides is serenity. I'm like the guy who has read the last chapter of a mystery book. I know how it all ends. So, even though there is pestilence and famine, even though there are wars and rumors of wars, I am comforted by the knowledge that everything works out the way God intends, and I can live with that, and so I can be serene amidst the chaos.

When you read this book, you may doubt my words. I know I will sound less than serene, because I felt less than serene. I can only say that, serenity is not always visible on the surface. During the months described in this book, I was like the guy who survived an earthquake. He's taken quite a beating, but he's alive. At the moment, however, he is trapped under tons of rubble. At some point in time, perhaps on this earth, perhaps in Heaven, God will remove all that rubble, and things will work out. So, I continue in my feeble efforts to follow God's will, and to praise Him with my life.

Most of the major events in the life of my family and myself are related in *Calvary's Child*, so I won't spend much time on that here. Instead, I will briefly cover the period of Carol's illness.

When Carol first started high school, she experienced respiratory troubles. Her family physician referred her to an asthma/allergy specialist, who diagnosed asthma. Carol first complained of stomach discomfort in the summer of 1993, when she was a rising high school senior. She saw a gastroenterologist, who ran a battery of tests. The results were negative. The doctor placed her on an antacid medication, assuming that she was experiencing digestive problems of some kind. In retrospect, I believe this was the cancer first making its presence known. There are many illnesses that manifest themselves as stomach discomfort, and small intestine cancer in an eighteen-year-old is so rare, no one even considered that possibility. Over the next several years, Carol complained off and on of stomach pain, but she did not seem to be in great discomfort. We continued to treat it as a minor inconvenience, like a headache. I spent some time doing research at the library on the Internet, but the focus of my research was in the area of ulcer diagnosis and treatment.

Carol suffered an increase in respiratory problems during her freshman year at High Point University. She made several trips to the emergency room and she spent several days in the hospital with pneumonia. Since she spent most of her time at High Point now, Carol located a family doctor there. He discovered that Carol was suffering from neutropenia, a blood disorder which results in a deficiency of neutrophils in the blood. Neutrophils help with the function of the immune system, and this disease often manifests itself in respiratory illnesses such as pneumonia. The doctor administered weekly shots, eventually restoring Carol's neutrophil levels to normal.

The doctor also discovered another problem. Carol had lupus, an autoimmune disease, which often results in causing a person's immune system to attack its own body. Symptoms include fatigue, muscle weakness, and sensitivity to light. In some cases, the disease will attack major organs such as the heart, brain, kidneys and lungs. It is likely that the lupus was the cause of Carol's neutropenia. Lupus also causes a diminished immune system. A properly functioning immune system is necessary for a person to fend off cancer. We all get cancer several times a year. In most cases, however, our immune systems kill the renegade cancer cells, and we remain healthy. In a few cases, the cancer cells gain a foothold and grow. The diminished immune systems of lupus sufferers make them more susceptible to the attacks of the cancer cells.

When a cancer cell gets a foothold, it begins to replicate. One cell becomes two. Two cells become four, and so on. In this manner, the initial growth of the cancer is relatively slow and almost always unnoticed. Only when the growth reaches a million cells or more is the cancer even remotely noticeable in a medical examination. By that time, the cancer's growth is exponential and rapid. One million cells become two million, and so on. By this time, the cancer is not easily overcome. Surgery is the preferred method, if all the cancer can be excised. Radiation and chemotherapy are used in addition to or instead of surgery, as appropriate.

In June of 1997, Carol's stomach discomfort grew dramatically worse. She complained of nausea after every meal. Before long, she was vomiting once a day, every day. By the end of July, her digestive system had stopped working completely. Early tests indicated that inflammation in the pylorus, where the stomach empties into the small intestine, had closed off the passage. Her doctors gave her medication, and performed a balloon procedure similar to that performed on heart patients. This was supposed to force an opening through the constricted area. It didn't work. In mid-August, Dr. Eisenhauer performed a gastric bypass operation. In this procedure he cut a new hole in the bottom of Carol's stomach, just above the blockage, and a new hole in the small intestine, just below the blockage. He then connected these two holes. The relief brought by this procedure was alarmingly brief.

On September 12, Dr. Eisenhauer operated again. This time he found the problem. The inflammation was actually a tumor. The tumor was inoperable because it had already surrounded a major artery in Carol's abdominal cavity, and it had already spread to the lining of the abdomen. Dr. William Medina entered the picture as Carol's oncologist. The first round of chemotherapy failed. Dr. Medina was considering a second round, although the outlook was pessimistic, when we decided to make the trip to Houston. M.D. Anderson is considered one of the two best cancer hospitals in the country. At M.D. Anderson, we met with Dr. Jaffer Ajani, one of the ten best gastroenterological oncologists in the world.

Our news was no better in Houston. Dr. Ajani concurred with Dr. Medina's recommended course of

7

chemotherapy, but cautioned us that this was only a "palliative" measure. Palliative is a fancy word, but according to Mr. Webster its definition is to, "lessen the pain or severity without actually curing."

In an oblique way, then, Dr. Ajani told us that Carol's condition was terminal. I think we realized that, particularly when Dr. Ajani offered no substantive alternatives, but we were not ready to acknowledge it. Upon our return to Hendersonville, we began the second round of chemotherapy.

At Christmas, Carol rallied long enough to make a trip to Mississippi to visit our family. That Carol was able to make this last trip was almost a miracle in itself. I think God gave her the strength to make the trip to say goodbye to all the Mississippi folks. Elaine also says it was miraculous that we were able to transport all the equipment that Carol needed. We own a GMC Jimmy SUV. When we make a trip to Mississippi, it is always full of clothes. At Christmas, it is also loaded with gifts. In addition to all this, we had to pack a gastric suction machine to keep Carol's stomach empty (which lessened her vomiting, but didn't eliminate it completely), and an enterol pump that pushed liquid nourishment through a tube into Carol's small intestine each night. Carol was fed with a tube which entered her stomach and passed through the bypass opening that Dr. Eisenhauer had made. Elaine claims that God made the space inside the Jimmy larger without making the outside dimensions larger. That may be. In any case, we made the trip.

After our return, Carol's condition declined rapidly. On January 16th, she entered the hospital, never to return home. On the night of January 17th, the hospital staff prepared us for her death. Nobody thought she would survive the night. She rallied however, and held on a little longer. I believe God left her here for another three weeks to allow Elaine and me to accept her death. While my head realized that, barring a miracle from God, she would not recover, my heart would not turn her loose. I could not conceive of living without my darling daughter.

During Carol's hospitalization, Elaine spent each night on a cot beside Carol's bed, while I slept at home. In the morning, I rose, dressed and rushed to the hospital to relieve Elaine, who went home, changed clothes and went to her teaching job at West Henderson High School. I stayed with Carol until 9:00, when a volunteer from our church arrived. Our church family really came through for us in this crisis. They helped us in so many ways – physically, emotionally and spiritually. At 9:00 I went to work and stayed until noon, when I rushed to the hospital for an hour. Another volunteer from the church arrived at 1:00 and stayed with Carol until 4:00, when I returned from work. Elaine went home from school, and returned to the hospital about 7:30 or so. And so, our life continued in a nightmarish blur.

Finishing school and getting her degree had been very important to Carol. When she was unsuccessful in her attempt to return to school in the fall of 1997, she was broken-hearted. She had completed all of her course work except for three semester hours. While Carol was still hospitalized in January, Dr. Vance Davis, High Point University's vice-president, called to report that the High Point's faculty and trustees had met and determined to award Carol the necessary three hours based on the extraordinary amount of extra-curricular work she had done. I was so happy for Carol I cried tears of joy. Carol was only semi-conscious. I told her again and again about the wonderful thing High Point had done. I am not sure if she ever understood completely. In Heaven now, I know she understands.

One afternoon, about a week before Carol died, I sat in the chair in her hospital room reading a Christian History magazine article about the Apostle Paul. The article quoted the following verse:

"Therefore we do not lose heart. Though outwardly we are wasting away, yet inwardly we are being renewed day by day. For our light and momentary troubles are achieving for us an eternal glory that far outweighs them all. So we fix our eyes not on what is seen, but on what is unseen. For what is seen is temporary, but what is unseen is eternal.. Now we know that if the earthly tent we live in is destroyed, we have a building from God, an eternal house in heaven, not built by human hands." II Corinthians 4:16 – 5:1.

My comprehension was just like the proverbial "light over the head" in a comic strip. Suddenly I understood what God had in store for Carol. This verse is often used in funeral services, and I know I had read or heard it many times, but this is the first time it really spoke to me. The treasure awaiting Carol in Heaven was so much greater than what she might encounter here on earth. God wasn't depriving Carol of any special privileges by taking her to Heaven early, she was just getting in on the "good stuff" ahead of us. For the first time, I felt as if I could let Carol go.

I wasn't dumb enough to think that losing Carol wouldn't be painful still. I knew I would have to grieve just as any person who loses a loved one. But I now believed that I would be able to release Carol without accusing God of being unfair, or blaming Him for depriving her of her life. I realized I had been too short-sighted in my view of what God had in store. It is kind of like driving a car. The idea is to look far down the road, to enable you to travel more safely, and to see your destination as soon as possible. If, on the other hand, you try to drive by focussing on your windshield, your trip will be unenjoyable and, probably, short. All you will see will be the bugs, dirt streaks and other grime stuck on the windshield. Following a practice like that will only make your trip harder, even if you avoid driving off in a ditch. You have to look beyond the windshield toward your destination. We Christians have to look beyond this physical life toward our Heavenly destination,

Carol's condition continued to deteriorate. She spent less and less time conscious. A parade of friends from High Point University, from West Henderson High School, and from church came by to share their love and concern and to pay their last respects.

On February 10th, I relieved the volunteer who sat with Carol at about 4:00. Carol had begun what is known as Cheyne-Stokes respiration, an erratic gasping breathing cycle. I didn't know it at the time, but it is an indicator of approaching death (but not a guarantee. Carol had exhibited this type of respiration the day after she was admitted to the hospital in January, but she recovered). I was exhausted. I sat in the reclining chair beside her bed and fell asleep within minutes. I didn't doze for long, ten or fifteen minutes, maybe. When I awoke, Carol had stopped breathing. Perhaps it was the cessation of her breathing that woke me. I buzzed for the nurse, who arrived to take her pulse and tell me what I already knew. Carol was dead.

CHAPTER TWO

"Not until the loom is silent and the shuttle ceases to fly
Shall God unfold the canvas and reveal the reasons why
The dark threads are as needful in the Weaver's skillful
hand
As the threads of gold and silver in the pattern He has
planned"
Barbara Johnson
Where Does a Mother Go to Resign?

Even our house seemed in shock the morning after Carol's death. I've never experienced such somber silence. The clocks refused to tick. The dishes wouldn't clatter. The walls couldn't echo. We were in a vacuum, which sucked away our very breath. Even as the stillness overwhelmed us, outpourings of love were rushing to fill that vacuum. Elaine's family was on its way from Mississippi and friends and loved ones were preparing messages of encouragement. Yet they hadn't had time to arrive.

Elaine and I arose and went about our morning activities as if in a nightmare. We may or may not have eaten breakfast. We may or may not have brushed our teeth. Who knows?

Larry Pace, a friend from the local computer club, rang our doorbell about midmorning. Five years earlier, Larry and Reisa had lost their seven-year-old son in a tragic accident. They were one of a few couples who knew what we were experiencing.

Larry gave us a book entitled *The Bereaved Parent* by Harriet Sarnoff Schiff. He told us that he and Reisa had gained some comfort from reading the book, and correctly surmised that it would help us. Over the next months,

Elaine and I read several books written by people who had lost children or other loved ones. They helped us endure our grief.

Larry offered words of comfort and encouragement. His presence reminded us that we could survive this loss, as unlikely as that prospect seemed at the moment.

"I believe your losing Carol may be more difficult that my loss," Larry said at one point. "Dean died quickly. You had to watch Carol fade away. I know that was a tremendous strain."

"You can't compare pain, Larry," I said. "We had a chance to prepare, at least a little bit, and to say goodbye. You didn't get that chance with Dean."

We agreed that both our losses were difficult. After a while Larry bade us goodbye, with a promise to see us later at the funeral home. A little over two years later, Larry succumbed to chronic lymphocytic leukemia and joined his son in Heaven. My heart still goes out to his widow Reisa and his daughter Julie.

Later that morning, Elaine and I drove to the funeral home to meet with Ron Shuler and plan Carol's funeral. Ron was very helpful and considerate, leading us through the decisions we needed to make. The previous night (Tuesday) we had decided to hold visitation at the funeral home on Wednesday night, and to hold the funeral at First Baptist Church on Thursday at 4:00. That really put Ron in a crunch. He barely made the newspaper deadline Tuesday night, a necessary step to inform those who wanted to make the visitation.

We had a reason, however. With so many relatives and loved ones in Mississippi who would be unable to make the trip to North Carolina, we planned a second service in Mississippi on Saturday. We needed Friday to make the five hundred-mile journey.

Months earlier, before Carol became sick, we had discussed the idea of funerals and burial arrangements in the abstract. On more than one occasion Carol had commented that her choice, when death came, would be cremation. Of course, none of us knew we would need to apply this choice so quickly. We had already decided to hold the funeral service at 4:00 on Thursday afternoon (to allow students and teachers from West Henderson High School to attend). Since Carol was to be cremated, we didn't need to plan an interment. We selected a casket designed for use in a cremation, and we brought the clothes for Carol to wear.

Carol wasn't a dress-up person. The most natural appearance for her would be casual. We brought her East Carolina University Medical School sweatshirt, to celebrate her acceptance into medical school and a High Point University baseball cap, to honor her role there. Jeans and tennis shoes completed the outfit.

After returning home to rest and allow Ron to prepare the body, we came back to the funeral home to have some time alone with Carol before visitation began.

I'm not sure who got the idea that somebody was supposed to look "natural" while lying in a casket. Please don't misunderstand, Ron did a great job. Carol lay peacefully in the casket with her arms folded across her waist. But she didn't look natural. Her ready smile was gone, and her eyes would never sparkle again.. We touched her cold hands and kissed her cold forehead. We knew, of course, that Carol was not in this body before us, she is in Heaven. But the sadness was still there. We stayed only a short while before heading back to our house

Not long before visitation, Elaine's family arrived from Mississippi. We greeted each other with hugs and tears. We were comforted by their presence. They helped with chores and judiciously inserted a little humor when our hearts got too heavy.

14

Shortly before 7:00 we made yet another trip to the funeral home. Ron displayed a couple of Carol's pictures in the chapel. One was of Carol when she was a young child, and one was a Glamour Shots portrait that Carol had used for her high school graduation. Ron had placed the pictures on either side of Carol's casket. The many flowers from friends and loved ones were arrayed around the room.

In her book *Grieving: How to Go on Living When Someone You Love Dies,* Dr. Teresa Rando emphasizes the importance of funeral rituals in the grieving process. I had lost loved ones before, but never had my heart been torn so deeply. I now understand how right Dr. Rando is.

At 7:00 Elaine and I lined up to the right of Carol's casket while Elaine's family lined up to the left. Visitors approached Elaine and me, then paused at the casket before proceeding to meet the others.

Whenever a family member of a friend or co-worker died, Elaine and I were conscientious about attending visitation at the funeral home or attending the funeral. We knew it was important to let them know that we cared, and that they were in our thoughts and prayers. For the next two hours, we received just such an outpouring.

I thought I had cried all my tears, but I had another supply somewhere. I heard that lack of rainfall had made the land overly dry. I was puzzled. I was sure Elaine and I had shed enough tears to flood the county. As one familiar face after another filed past, as one person after another hugged me, I washed their cheeks and shoulders with my tears. I was comforted by the love of those who helped us remember Carol.

The First Baptist Church choir ended practice early to attend the visitation. A busload of students and professors from High Point University made the trip. One of those who came was Dr. Charlie Warde, Carol's Irish chemistry professor. When he reached the end of the hand-shaking

15

journey along the line of Elaine's four sisters and two brothers, he stopped. Puzzled, he asked, "Are you Catholic?" No, he was assured, we're just a large family. By 9:00 the line had dwindled, and it was time for visitation to end. Our hearts were warmed by the demonstration of affection from so many people.

The Bereavement Committee at FBC provided lunch for us the next day. We drove to the church, where the committee had arranged tables and place-settings. We sat, and the committee served, keeping our plates and glasses filled. Elaine's family remarked time and again how warm and solicitous our church family was.

As the afternoon waned, we dressed for the funeral. Ron Shuler brought a limousine and carried us from our house to the church. We had scheduled the service for 4:00 to allow any teachers and students from West Henderson High School to attend.

Suzy Waldrop graciously played the organ for the ceremony. Skip Fendley sang a couple of beautiful songs. Brother Steve Scoggins followed with a message. Here are some excerpts:

"Tom and Elaine and family, we want you to know that we love you, and we've been praying for you. Everyone is here today because they want you to know that we are going to stand by you. We are here today because we love Carol. What a sweet, Christian girl! She touched so many lives, and I count it an honor to say that I got to know her, that she was my friend. I think the fact that she touched lives can be seen. We've got two busses from High Point. We've got folks from Appalachian State University, we've got folks from Mississippi. She touched a lot of lives.

"God put two passages on my heart. One is II Timothy 4. Paul says, 'I have fought the good fight. I have finished the race. I have kept the faith. Now there is in store for me the crown of righteousness, which the Lord, the righteous

Judge will award to me on that day – not only me, but also to all who have longed for His appearing.'

"Elaine, I think you were in the room a couple of nights ago when I shared with you, that girl is walking into a bunch of reward. I believe she is receiving a crown. She's in heaven, of course, but I think she's going to have a bountiful reward. One other passage that just has to be read today. In fact, Jim handed me the copy that you printed and put on the hospital room wall, because this verse meant so much to you. II Corinthians 4:16 and following. 'Therefore, we do not lose heart, though outwardly we are wasting away, yet inwardly we are being renewed day by day. For our light and momentary troubles are achieving for us an eternal glory that far outweighs them all. So, we fix our eyes not on what is seen, but on what is unseen. For what is seen is temporary and what is unseen is eternal.'

"Let's pray. Lord, I come to you now, and I thank you that you're here. We don't have to beg for your presence. You said, 'I will never leave you nor forsake you.' And Father, I've seen your grace uphold Tom and Elaine. I've seen you give them a peace when their strength had run out. I thank you for that. I claim now, Lord, the strength and the grace which will be sufficient for tomorrow, and for next month and for next year. Father, I thank you for how strong you were in Carol's life. I thank you for her witness. I thank you for the people she led to you. I thank you for the testimony she gave, Lord. I thank you that with my own eyes, I watched as you gave her such grace in her sickness. So God of grace, we come to you now. We come to the throne of grace, and we ask you to bring your comfort to every heart here. In Jesus' name, amen."

"Paul said, 'I fought the good fight. I finished my race. I kept the faith.' Carol could have said that. I watched this sweet girl as she grew up. I watched this sweet girl as she went to college. She lived for Jesus in high school, brought

17

Campus Crusade for Christ to High Point University. She fought a good fight. But I also want to tell you she finished her race. Tom and I were talking a while back, and the one thing that that I think has gripped my heart about Carol's life is this: she probably did more in 21 – almost 22 years than most do in 70. She touched more lives in that amount of time than most do in 70 years. But I want you to know her race was only to be this long. She finished it. I meet very few people who finish the task God gives them. Carol finished her race. Paul also said, Not only did I fight the good fight, I ran my race. He said, I kept the faith.

"I've noticed through the years that if you want to know what someone is really like, you must see them in weakness and you must see them in sickness. I've become so impressed with Tom and Elaine, as I've seen their strength. But I'll guarantee you this. If anyone doubted that Carol was real, they just haven't been around her in the last few weeks. Don't get around me if I get sick, you won't find the same thing! She was always sweet. She never got angry. She didn't get aggravated. She was always so kind. She ministered to the nurses. She'd look up, sometimes she'd just barely be able to keep her eyes open for a minute. But she'd say, 'Would you give me a hug?' She talked about her love for the Lord. I want to tell you something, when you're that low you can't fake it! It was real in her. She could say, 'I kept the faith.'

"Now, with all that said about Carol, we need to say, 'What about us today?'

"Tom, I want to take the verse that God gave you, and I want to use it as the theme for the few thoughts I want to give.

"'So we fix our eyes not on what is seen, but on what is unseen.' The verse that Paul puts here says we have to change the way we look at things. Tom and Elaine, you don't know how many people have come up and said, 'You

18

better pray for me on this one. I'm struggling with this. I'm going to have a talk with God on this.' We have a whole church that's hurting. We share the pain that you share.

"But I want to share three ways to look at this differently. Number one, we look not on what is seen, but what is unseen. Number two, we've got to focus not on the questions we don't have an answer for, we have to focus on trusting God. I've had many a person in our church come and say, 'Pastor, why is this happening? Why Carol, of all folks? Why so young?'

"I wish I could give you an answer, but I don't have one. I can tell you this, God is still in control. Jesus is risen. Heaven is real. Grace is still sufficient.

"There are questions we'll never have an answer for in this life. One day we'll get to heaven and we'll figure it out. We'll say, 'God, that's what you were up to! But right now, instead of focussing on the questions we don't have an answer for, we have to focus on putting faith in God. You know as a parent. I know as a parent, kids go through this "why" stage. Do you remember that, when they are real little? They come up to you and say, 'Why, Daddy? Why this and why that?' I said I would always be a patient father, who would sit down and explain it all. But my children know that didn't happen. There were times I just looked at them and said, 'Trust me.'

"How can you explain it to a two year old? I think there is a sense in which all of us have to come at time to God and say, 'God, why?' God has to say, 'trust me.' Because there is no way our little minds can understand God's plans. We have to change our focus from the questions we have to the God we trust.

"Second, there is a temptation to focus on the years that you'll be apart. But I want to encourage you to focus on the years you've had together. You folks were blessed. I know it's been tough, but if you could go back and say 'I'd just as soon not have children', you would never say that. You wouldn't give anything for these 21 years would you? You were so blessed by God. I thought, my soul, you folks have shed tears. You've gone through the heartaches. But I could point out parents – I'm not going to – whose children are the same age and they've shed tears, and they've had sleepless nights, and they've been afraid the phone would ring. Because they've had children who gave them such heartaches. You never had to hang your head in shame about Carol, did you? You never had to worry, I wonder where she is? You knew she was at a Bible study somewhere. You didn't have to wonder if she was going to fail. She was one of the best students anybody ever had. You had a daughter who blessed you for 21 years. You had a daughter who honored you for 21 years. You will be tempted to sit here, year after year, counting how many years you are apart. I want to encourage you, instead, to focus on the years you were together. Then you can sing what Skip sang. Now you can give thanks with a grateful heart.

"Lastly, this verse says, don't look at what is seen, look at what is unseen. The third thing we have to do is we have to change our focus – instead of looking at this world, we have to focus on Heaven. If I could, I would pull the curtain back and let us see her. That was a sweet girl. She glowed. She had the joy of the Lord. But if you could see her now, you'd hardly recognize her. She knows more joy than she ever knew at High Point. She knows more joy than she ever knew at West High. She glows right now! The one thing we have to do is remember that this (knocking on pulpit) is temporary, and that (pointing to Heaven) is eternal. I know this for a fact. Starting two days ago, Heaven became a lot more real to you. Heaven became a lot more precious to you. When D.L. Moody was dying –

he'd had a heart attack – his son came to see him. He said, 'Dad, I want to pray that God will heal you.' D.L. Moody answered, 'I don't want that. So much that I love is over there (Heaven) now.' Right now you could say that. It's not hard to obey Colossians 3, which says set you heart on things above. So much of your heart is there now.

"'Therefore we do not lose heart.' Tom, that was the word God gave you. That's the word that got you and Elaine through these last few weeks. And that's going to be the word that six months from now, 2 years from now, still going to be the word that God's going to give you.

"Let's pray. Oh, Father, you promised us that when we were weak, you'd send your strength and we'd be strong. We feel weak today. I pray that your comfort would flood hearts. I thank you that we are here today, and the tears are for us because we are going to miss Carol. But there's no tear being shed because anyone has a doubt about whether or not Carol is in heaven. Lord Jesus, You took those angels into her room. You took her into your presence, and she is there and we praise You for that. I pray now in the name of Jesus, that all of us who get so caught up in the world will this afternoon look on what is unseen. Let Heaven become real to everyone. In Jesus' name, Amen."

21

CHAPTER THREE

As the service continued, Brother Jim Pearce, who had served as Carol's youth minister offered some words about her life:

"Tom and Elaine, first I want to thank you for the privilege of sharing a few words about a special friend of mine and of ours – Amanda Carol Hooker. I've entitled my thoughts, 'Somebody I'll Never Forget.'

"I got that title from one of the nurses who stood over her bed Tuesday night. She said, 'I'll never forget Carol.' And she started to cry. 'I'll never forget the impact she had on my life in this last month. I will never be the same.'

"Those are powerful words from a professional who works on an oncology ward and watches people die, if not daily at least weekly. To say, '"My life will never be the same. I'm thankful I knew Carol.'

"Philippians Chapter One says, 'For what is life? To me, it is Christ. Death then, will be more.' When I think of Carol, I think that verse sums up her life. What is life? It is Christ. It's exciting to see that, as we think about Carol's life, she wasn't just some little saint that floated around. Steve was talking about what a sweet kid she was.

"When the Hookers moved here in 1988 from Mississippi, Carol was a different person. I don't think she really wanted to move here. And the Carol that I first got to know was *mean.* In fact, until a bout a year ago, I kept two black gloves that Carol used to wear. You know, the ones with the fingers out of them. She used to wear that kind of stuff. I can remember that Carol would get so angry that she would go into the gym down here, and she would punch the walls until her hands were bloody. She was angry. But praise God, to watch the change, as Jesus Christ became

22

more real in her. We come here today not so much to praise Carol, but to praise Jesus who made Carol what she was.

"It would be so easy for us to say, 'My, what a sweet girl, I wish we could be like Carol.' Guess what? We can. The power of God's spirit lives in you, and the power of God's spirit lives in me. We can be like Carol, because Carol strove to be like Jesus. To live is Christ. Tom and I were cutting up in the hospital room one day, because Carol didn't really like being in that bed at all. Several times she would say, 'Let's go! Let's go! Get my clothes, we're going.'

"'Where are we going?'

"'We're gonna go eat jambalaya!'

"Guess what? She's having a Cajun feast. I'm so thankful for Carol. When I think about Carol, I think back to that seventh grader, but then I watched as God took hold of her life. I watched as God put many of you into her life to build her into who she was. I think of Glenda Lancaster and the strategic role that Glenda played as the guidance counselor at Rugby Junior High. Glenda reminded me recently that Carol was one of the ones who started the club Rugby Against Drugs and was part of the national organization PRIDE. She went to Houston Texas to speak at the national convention. See, one of the things that encouraged me about Carol, she wasn't just a Jesus freak. She was involved in all aspects of her community, and with people.

"I'm thankful for Carol. I think of Carol as the first one on the bus, who always wanted to go to the prisons. I've watched 150 mean men stilled to the drop of a needle as Carol stood in boldness and talked about Jesus. That was the Carol that we remember.

"I think of Carol on mission trips, boldly walking up to people that no one else would approach and sharing her faith with them, being a friend to them. Carol cared about

23

people, and that caring developed as her life developed. She got a burden for her classmates and for her professors at High Point University. She helped lead four of her professors to know Christ as their Savior. She helped start the Campus Crusade movement at High Point University. That wasn't an easy task. Sometimes when you try to do something new, it doesn't go over well. But she and her friends, some of whom are sitting here today, said we are going to stick it out because we believe Jesus wants to be seen through this organization we call Campus Crusade for Christ.

"Carol was bold. I talked to one of Carol's dear friends the other night, a person she got to know through Disciple Now since he came to do the music – Sal Oliveri. Sal cried on the phone. He said, 'I wish I could be there, Jim. There's no way I can get out of my commitments. But I want you to know, when I came to Disciple Now that last time and I heard her give her testimony, I wept. I've never seen that kind of passionate love in somebody for Jesus.'

"Wherever she went, there was something of the aroma of Christ, the scripture says, that trailed behind her. That attracted people to her. I remember Tima (Duncan) telling me a funny story. By the way, Tima probably spent more time in the hospital than anybody else. I'd go in her room and find Tima stroking her hand, or I'd find Denise Berry rubbing oil on her feet to keep her skin from cracking. So many loving people gathered around her. But Tima said that she and Christopher Smith were on a retreat one time, counseling her. If you've ever counseled a young person, sometimes counseling a young person is like counseling this pulpit here, 'No!'

"They just poured their hearts out. They said everything they could say. 'Are you going to get right with Jesus?' Of course, expecting her to say no. She said, 'Yes, now. I'm going to do it.' Their jaws dropped. She said,

'Let's do it. Now. Let's get busy. Let's make this straight.' Something I admired about Carol was her honesty. She was hot or cold – never in between. She was yes or she was no. I pray that my life could be a yes or a no more than an in-between. Maybe some of us are in-betweens. Carol was not.

"One of the most powerful things I've heard in the last couple of days was when Trent and Marianna Dollyhigh came to me last night and said that their lives had been so impacted by Amanda Carol Hooker that when they have a daughter, they are going to call her Carol. That says a lot, it says a lot about the Jesus they saw in Carol.

"So again, we are reminded, why was Carol such a special person? Well, to live is Christ. She allowed Jesus Christ to live through her. She wasn't perfect, but she was available to God, and she was available to others. I don't think I've ever been so impressed with a young person as when I watched Carol go through her high school years. God by His Spirit began to convict her that she was rebelling against her parents. Maybe not outwardly, but inwardly. I remember the day when Carol said, 'From now on, I am going to submit to my parents. I don't care what they say.' Several of you who knew Carol can remember with dumbfoundment as you watched her submit to her parents. And you said, 'how can she do that?' It was the Spirit of Jesus. You see, Carol believed that her God was big enough that if He wanted her to be able to do a certain thing, He would change their hearts instead of her having to manipulate them to get what she wanted. I can remember the last two years at high school, she didn't do anything unless she had her parents blessing. There were times when Tom said, 'Well, if you really want to do that, you can do it, but I don't really like it.'

"Carol said, 'If you are not 100%, I'm not doing it' That's the Spirit of Jesus.

"I had lunch today with one of Carol's friends. Meghan reminded me of a beautiful illustration. People come in and out of our lives and we don't really understand why they are there at the time. But as we look back in hindsight, we can see how God used them to steer us more toward Jesus. When you think of Amanda Carol Hooker, every one of us here can remember that, because her life touched ours for a brief while, we were directed more toward Jesus Christ and more toward His cross. No greater thing can be said, Tom and Elaine, than that a person was pointed toward Jesus Christ because of a life. And that's what Carol did for me, and for us. Let's pray together.

"Father we are so thankful that we had the brief privilege to know Carol. I know I'll never be the same because of that. Many here would say the same. Father, I pray for myself and for each one of us here that we would learn from her life. What it means to be sold out to Jesus. And what good things happen when you're sold out. It doesn't mean that there's not going to be any more pain, no more disease. But people being led to what is eternal. Lord, thank you for Carol's life. God, I pray that for each person here you would encourage us to look toward the eternal. Move toward the unseen. Someday, when our time comes, people would be able to say of us, Philippians 1:21. To live is Christ. In the name of Christ we pray, amen."

Afterwards, we invited the High Point University bunch to the house to help eat the food brought by so many friends. When they had gone, Larry McCord and I went downstairs for a few minutes of quiet. We spoke about Carol's life, and touched on what might have been.

"This means that now I'll never have grandchildren." I said.

Poor Larry! How was this man, who was a grandfather several times over, supposed to respond to that? Actually, he recovered very well.

26

"I'll let you have one of mine," he said. He didn't tell me which one he was offering, though! That touch of humor helped me through at least one melancholy moment.

The following day we loaded our cars and headed for Mississippi. We packed the pictures of Carol to display at the church, and we packed some of the flowers, as well.

The memorial service at Ellistown Baptist Church was scheduled for Saturday morning. Brother Leland Hogan, our pastor from Carterville Baptist Church made the 250-mile journey to Ellistown for the service. Here are some excerpts from his remarks:

"I count it a privilege and an honor to stand with the Hooker family in memory of Carol, a very precious young lady that I got to know some years ago as her pastor at Carterville Baptist Church in Petal. There is a poem that describes a little girl. This little girl is down on the seashore. She has built a sandcastle. As the waves begin to wash against the shore, and the tide begins to rise, the water washes away her sandcastle. She goes to her mother. She cries because her sandcastle has been washed away. Her mother says to her, 'Hush, child. For the waves that have washed away your sandcastle are the waves that will bring your father home.'

"In our lives there are events that wash away something that is very precious to us. But at the same time, it brings a greater victory. And though we come this morning remembering a person who is no longer with us physically, we rejoice at what God has done in her life, and we praise Him for it. I have not come to grieve with you, but I have come to rejoice with you in reality, claiming the praise that the Lord gave to us when He said, 'Blessed are those that mourn, for they shall be comforted.'

"We rejoice in that. And we rejoice in the fact that Jesus Christ gave His life that we might have life. We rejoice in all that God does for us, and so it is my prayer today that we might rejoice in the life that Carol lived. We might rejoice in her contribution to the world, in the years that God gave her to us, and we might remember her fondly.

"I want to read a passage from the book of Joshua. Chapter four, verse nine says, 'Joshua set up the twelve stones that had been in the middle of the Jordan at the spot where the priests who carried the Ark of the Covenant had stood. And they are there to this day.'

"Let me share the picture here. The children of Israel had wandered in the wilderness for forty years. Moses was dead. Joshua had come to the place of leadership. God is now ready to move the people forward into the Promised Land. They encamped at a place known as the Grove of the Acacia trees. God spoke to Joshua and said to him, 'Move the people forward to the Jordan River.' The Jordan river was overflowing its banks. The children of Israel did not lose faith. but surely they wondered, 'How will we move over this Jordan?' You know, there are many Jordans in our lives. Many obstacles that come to us that we don't understand how we are going to get through them. I'm sure that in the days past for some members of Carol's family there have been those Jordans that seem impossible to cross.

"God said to Joshua, 'The people need to be reminded of what happened on this occasion. Pick one man from each tribe to select a stone from the bed of the Jordan River and carry it to the other side. There build a memorial that will speak to the lives of the future generations of how great God is.' Why? God wanted the people of Israel to remember that He was present in their lives.

"When the word came to us of Carol's death, and I sat down with these verses of scripture, I began to think of Carol and her life. I began to think of the memorial that she has given us, a life that we can look upon and recall pleasant memories. I remembered her younger years. When I first got to know Carol she was about six years old.

I saw in her life a memorial. Things that will bring joy to our hearts in days to come. I thought about the time when she was born. When this precious baby was given to Tom and Elaine by God. How Carol was held in their arms. A memorial stone in her life.

"I'm sure that Tom and Elaine remember the time when she took her first step. This is always a monumental time in the life of a child. We then have to follow closely behind her to pick up what she's pulled off the shelves. A memorial stone.

"When she started her first day of school. This is always a traumatic time in the life of a parent. We have to turn them loose a little bit. Another stone of memory.

"There were those times when she began to ask about Jesus Christ. Those times when she was concerned about her own salvation. And the time when she came to know Christ as Lord of her life.

"We would not forget the time when she got her driver's license. In the lives of parents, that certainly is a scary moment. We are glad because we don't have to carry her so many places, and yet we are sad because we have to stay up and wait until she gets in. A memorial stone.

"It was exciting when she was accepted into medical school, and would have begun this fall. It says something of her mentality – of her intellect. I remember the time when I used to give Elaine fits. I prodded her and told her that women were just not as smart in math as men were (laughter). Carol was a young lady with a great deal of intelligence. Another memorial stone in her monument.

"There were some other things that were important in her life. Carol was committed to her church at Carterville. As we followed her family through their lives at Hendersonville, she was committed to her church. She was God's person. This is probably one of the larger stones in her monument.

29

"She had a concern for children because she loved to witness for Christ. She witnessed for Christ as a child, she witnessed for Christ as a young person. She wanted to do some things in school that were not permissible because of the laws of our land today.

"Friends were important to her. People were important to her. And yet her love for you – her family and friends was important in her life.

"And so Carol has placed these stones to build her monument, stones that we will remember for the rest of our lives. There is one other thing I want to share about her. Carol's life was in order when God came to get her. On top of this monument is the biggest stone of all – her house was in order. She had made it right with God."

Several members of Elaine's family and mine had concerns about our decision to cremate Carol. That is a practice that had never been followed by anyone in either family. Of course, the question of having a body in Heaven after the rapture was not a factor. God can reconstitute the body from anything or nothing. I think the concern was the break with tradition and the fact that there would be no gravesite to visit.

We addressed one of those issues. We selected a plot in the Ellistown Cemetery. We put a headstone at the plot and listed all three of our names. We decided to go a little further, we decided that we could store the container with Carol's ashes inside the headstone. That would give everyone, including us, a place to visit and put flowers. We would also have a resting place for ourselves when the time came.

After the service, we traveled to Mom and Dad's home. I hadn't seen Dad since his surgery. When we entered the house, he began crying. I had seen my father cry so few times, and my emotional condition was so raw, I didn't really know what to do. I was unable to comfort him, and he was unable to comfort Elaine and me.

I had told Mother and Pam not to come to North Carolina for the funeral there. I knew they needed to be available to take care of Daddy. I also know that not being with us in North Carolina was difficult for them and for Daddy, too. They have always been ready, willing and able to do anything that we needed.

On Sunday morning, we rose early and made the 500 mile trip back to North Carolina. Carol died on Tuesday, we planned the funeral and held visitation on Wednesday, held the funeral on Thursday, drove 500 miles on Friday, held another funeral on Saturday, and drove 500 miles on Sunday. We did all this so we could go back to work on Monday! In retrospect we did too much.

God's Loan

"I'll lend to you, for a little time
A child of mine," He said.
"For you to love the while she lives
and mourn for when she's dead."

"It may be six or seven years,
or twenty-two or three.
But will you 'til I call her back,
Take care of her for me?"

"She'll bring her charms to gladden you,
and should her stay be brief,
you'll have these precious memories,
as solace for your grief."

31

"I cannot promise she will stay,
since all from Earth return.
But there are lessons taught down there
I want this child to learn."

"I've looked this whole world over
in my search for teachers true,
and in the crowds that throng life's land
I have selected you."

"Now will you give her all your love,
not think the labor vain,
nor hate Me when I come to call
to take her back again?"

It seems to me, I heard them say,
"Dear Lord, Thy will be done.
For all the joys Thy child shall bring,
The risk of grief we'll run."

"We'll shelter her with tenderness.
We'll love her while we may,
And for the happiness we've known,
Forever grateful stay."

"And should the angels call for her
much sooner than we'd planned,
we'll brave the bitter grief that comes
and try to understand."
Barbara Johnson, *Where Does a Mother Go to Resign?*

CHAPTER FOUR

"After Nathan had gone home, the Lord struck the child that Uriah's wife had borne to David, and he became ill. David pleaded with God for the child. He fasted and went into his house and spent the nights lying on the ground. The elders of his household stood before him to get him up from the ground, but he refused and he would not eat any food with them.

"On the seventh day, the child died. David's servants were afraid to tell him that the child was dead for the thought, 'While the child was still living, we spoke to David but he would not listen to us. How can we tell him that the child is dead? He may do something desperate.'

"David noticed that his servants were whispering among themselves, and he realized the child was dead. 'Is the child dead?' He asked.

"' Yes', they replied. 'He is dead.'

"Then David got up from the ground. After he had washed, put on lotions and changed his clothes, he went into the house of the Lord and worshipped. Then he went to his own house, and at his request, they served him food, and he ate.

"His servants asked him, "Why are you acting this way? While the child was alive, you fasted and wept, but now that the child is dead, you get up and eat!'

"He answered, 'While the child was still alive, I fasted and wept. I thought, 'Who know, the Lord may be gracious to me and let the child live.' But now that he is dead, why should I fast? Can I bring

him back again? I will go to him, but he will not
return to me.'"

II Samuel 12:15-23

David's strength amazes me. I've learned how difficult
it is to lose a child. For David to return to "normal" life so
quickly is a testament to the strength of his character. I
suspect, however, that David's heart was laden with pain for
his child, and I believe he may have disguised his true
feelings for the sake of his wife and his household.

I was unable to display that kind of strength. Already
physically and emotionally exhausted from standing by
Carol during her illness, I returned to work out of a sense of
obligation because we were so shorthanded. I knew the
office could not afford to be short another person.

It was almost my undoing. I was tired when I crawled
out of bed in the morning. By mid-day, I was practically
worthless. My senses were numb. My head felt as if it
were filled with mud. Thinking coherently was impossible.
Mercifully, my co-workers avoided burdening me with any
unnecessary tasks, and I muddled through each day as best I
could. When I arrived home in the afternoons, I collapsed
onto the couch and tried to sleep off my perpetual headache.

Our friends, co-workers and church family still carried
us in their hearts. Over the next several weeks we received
many thoughtful cards and notes. For example:

> "At the same time I grieve with you and Elaine,
> yet we join you in praising God for the blessing she
> has been. I look forward to meeting her in the
> resurrection." Buddy Coiner, Columbus GA.

> "I thank God for the privilege of knowing your
> daughter. She was a fine person in every way. I am
> sure that theses past several months have been most
> agonizing for you and for Carol. Yet, I am just as

confident that you are thankful for the Christ in whom Carol placed her abiding trust." Dr. Robert E. Williams, Pastor, Parkwood Baptist Church, High Point NC.

"My thoughts are still with you because I know it takes time – and time with God – 'Keep looking up'. Jesus loves you." Lula Mae Briggs, Hendersonville NC

"The Wednesday night after Carol died we were in choir practice singing 'In the Presence of Jehovah', when Gwen Perkins turned to me and said, 'that's where Carol Hooker is now, and I bet it's great.' The more I've thought about that, the more I've realized that it is indeed great to know that Carol is in the presence of her Maker and that she influenced others while on this earth that they too might one day be in the presence of Jehovah." Rose Rainey, Petal MS.

"Carol truly touched our hearts. Ruth Ann introduced us to her as a dear friend at High Point University. One time Carol was experiencing a troubled time with her health and Ruth Ann called me and we put her on our prayer list as church. When Carol found this out she wrote me the sweetest note of appreciation. I still have that note.

"Carol was a true friend to our daughter and we will never forget her for her generosity of friendship to Ruth Ann.

"Just think, she is in the arms of her precious Lord, no longer in pain. We rejoice for the testimony that she has left behind.' Richard & Kay Milam, Elkview WV.

"It is my prayer that you have had some time to rest over the past few days. I know the previous months and especially the last few weeks have been very difficult for you. We continue to pray that the presence and peace of our Lord will sustain you in the days ahead.

"Carol was a flower among the thorns. In the face of all the worldly peer pressure she remained faithful in her testimony for Jesus. Only God knows how many lives were and will be changed by her strong commitment." Rev. Leland Hogan, Carterville Baptist Church, Petal Ms.

"I hope you know that I, along with so many others, have been thinking of and praying for you, Elaine and Carol for quite some time now and will continue to do so. It's never easy to give up someone so dear as I know Carol was to you. When Dad died this past June, it was tough to give him up and not want him with us, but it was also good to know he could once again be the wonderful, joyful and fun-loving person he was before he became so sick and burdened with his heart problems. Joe, Pam, Shauna and Josh Sewell, The Colony TX.

"My heart is heavy for you. The journey you have begun is a long one. Grieving is a <u>long hard</u> process. But I can promise you one thing. God will be there for you, whether you can feel Him or not. For a long time after we lost Hannah, I didn't feel anything. A numbness set in, I guess. Looking back, I know He was there, sustaining me through every single minute. That the only explanation I have for how I made it through the long, dark tunnel I found myself in. At the end, He was the light." Wanda Reynolds, Petal MS.

"Everyone wishes that you wouldn't have to go through this and that Carol could have lived, but that is our human way of looking at the situation.

Your Christian friends know that it is all in God's plan and that he will bring you through stronger and certainly Carol is experiencing great comfort and joy." Tom & Carol Hardesty, Bluffton SC.

"I can't imagine the sorrow you are facing right now. Just know that you are admired for finishing your job well – not many people will ever have a child who turned out as beautifully as Carol did. So many people will be influenced by her life and character. You both are greatly respected by all of us." Pat Worsham, Hendersonville NC.

I continued to struggle with denial. The reality of my life was enshrouded in a sense of unreality. I could not believe that Carol was gone. I knew my mind carried many happy memories of Carol and our times together, but those memories were locked away in a closet in the back of my mind, and I couldn't find the key. My mind kept flashing back to a vision of Carol's lifeless body on the hospital bed. And yet, even that memory was too painful for me to tolerate for more than a second or two. It was like grabbing a hot skillet. As soon as my mind touched that memory, it flinched and turned away.

In fact, all my senses were in a state of shock. My numbness – my sense of unreality was God's insulation from the pain of my grief. It was like wearing an oven mitt to hold that hot skillet. While wearing an oven mitt, a cook's sense of touch is diminished. But that is the only way she can hold the skillet without being severely burned. It provides a layer of insulation to protect her from the pain.

God had encased my senses in an oven mitt, providing a layer of insulation to protect me from the pain of my loss. Yet it diminished my senses, and I struggled to function.

The renowned Christian author C.S. Lewis lost his wife, Joy, to cancer late in his life. He wrote a book entitled *A*

Grief Observed, which is really a journal of the grief he experienced after her death. Here are some excerpts from that book:

"No one ever told me that grief felt so like fear. I am not afraid, but the sensation is like being afraid. The same fluttering in the stomach, the same restlessness, the yawning. I keep swallowing.

"At other times it feels like being mildly drunk, or concussed. There is a sort of invisible blanket between the world and me. I find it hard to take in what anyone says, Or perhaps, hard to want to take it in. It is so uninteresting. Yet I want the others to be about me. I dread the moments when the house is empty. If only they would talk to one another and not to me.

"An no one told me about the laziness of grief...I loathe the slightest effort. Not only writing, but even reading a letter is too much...only as a dog tired man wants an extra blanket on a cold night; he'd rather lie there shivering than get up and find one.

"One never meets just cancer, or war, or unhappiness (or happiness). One only meets each hour or moment that comes. All manner of ups and downs. Many bad spots in our best times, many good ones in our worst.

"You never know how much you really believe anything until its truth or falsehood becomes a matter of life and death to you. It is easy to say you believe a rope to be strong and sound as long as you are merely using it to cord a box. But suppose you had to hang by that rope over a precipice? Wouldn't you then first discover how much you really trusted it?

"Aren't all these notes the senseless writings of a man who won't accept the fact that there is nothing we can do with suffering except to suffer it?

"What do people mean when they say, "I am not afraid of God because I know He is good?" Have they never been to a dentist?"

Stresses at work compounded my difficulties. We were shorthanded, and our always busy office was stretched to the breaking point. Additionally, we were adding new technology which would help us in the long run. In the short run, however, it impaired our efficiency even more.

During much of the December before Carol's death, we wired our office for the installation of modular furniture. At the time we had a large open office, with the employees desks distributed across the space in rank and file fashion. The open space robbed our claimants of privacy during their claims interviews and resulted in a noisy, hectic work environment.

The modular furniture provided a cubicle for each employee. Scott Adams, who draws the "Dilbert" comic strip, pokes fun at the cubicle as a workplace environment. Actually, it provides a quieter, more private space for the employee to work. We looked forward to it.

The preparatory work required extra time from me. I had to be on hand during "off hours" so the electricians could install the wiring and circuits for the modules, and so they could "pull the cables", running data cables from the computer room through the ceiling space to the location of each module. Once the furniture modules were installed, our computer terminals would be hooked to these cables.

Now, I found myself rushing back to work the week after Carol's death. I reported to work on Monday morning after planning and attending two memorial services and driving one thousand miles in only a few days. I did it because I believed the office couldn't afford to be without me. In truth, my ability to contribute was very small. I could very well have precipitated a collapse of my own, and

I very nearly did. I would have done better to rest for another week, or at least a couple of days.

In *Grieving: How to Go On Living When Someone You Love Dies,* Dr. Terese Rando says, "The death of your child exposes you to the most intense, complicated and long-lasting grief known to humans."

On top of all of this, my father's condition worsened. I was 500 miles from him, and my mother and her sisters were the ones most involved in caring for his needs, but I still felt the concern for his condition as much as my muddled senses would allow.

Daddy was seventy-five years old. He was born in Pontotoc County in 1922, and except for the time he was in military service and the time he was in the Civilian Conservation Corps, he lived all his years there. The first years of his life were spent on the farm that his parents, Stanford and Lillie Mae Hooker rented just west of Pontotoc on Highway 336. This farm was just west of the "channel", perhaps four miles out of town. In 1929, Stanford bought a place a little further west, in the community of Thaxton. Daddy graduated from Thaxton High School as valedictorian of his graduating class.

He joined the Marine Corps in 1943, and served as a regimental radio operator in the Pacific Theater. He served on Hawaii, the Johnston Islands, and Palau during his active duty. Upon his return from the Marines, he married Bernette Coleman.

He and my mother built a small house beside his parents and he began his routine of helping operate the farm. They planted cotton as a cash crop. In addition they planted corn for the few head of cows, peanuts, popcorn, and sweet potatoes. Mother and grandmother contributed by helping hoe and pick the cotton, milk the cows, and tend the garden, which included sweet corn, tomatoes, butter beans, green beans, peas, and Irish potatoes (plus some stuff

I don't remember, I'm sure). In addition, the farm yielded Muscatine grapes (for jelly) apples, figs, pecans and walnuts. My parents were able to produce almost everything they needed to live on right on the farm.

Daddy really didn't care much for the farming life. In the late 1950's when my sister Pam and I started school, he went to work for his cousin, Oakley Hooker, as a carpenter. About that time, Mother started work in the shirt factory in Pontotoc. So we made the transition from a farm family to a 'rural" family, one which lived in the country, but did not earn its living from farming. I think Daddy was much happier after that. He also became known as a "jack-of-all-trades". He used the skills he learned as a radio operator to repair radios and (later) televisions in the community. When solid state circuitry replaced the vacuum tube, however, he considered himself "oboslete" and gave up that skill. People in the community also often called upon Daddy to repair such appliances as ovens, washers and dryers. He did his own repairs on the automobiles he owned until technology made those too complicated, as well.

In 1997, Daddy began having physical problems. During one physical exam, a chest X-ray found a spot on his lung. The doctor recommended that Dad's right lung be removed. That was done in January 1998, shortly before Carol died. Follow-ups on the surgery revealed that the cancer had metastasized. He went to an oncologist, who administered chemotherapy. By the end of April, however, we learned that the chemo had not stopped the cancer, and that Daddy's condition was terminal. Our beleaguered family faced another illness and apparently, another death.

Daddy took the news very well. As a Christian, he knew where he was going. He had lived a long life, and realized that death comes to us all sooner or later. I am sure he did not prefer this path, but he accepted it with

41

equanimity. Hospice took over responsibility for his care, and nurses there provided for pain medication and worked with Mom to help make Dad as comfortable as possible.

CHAPTER FIVE

I am poured out like water,
All my bones are out of joint.
My heart has turned to wax;
It has melted away within me.
                    Psalm 22:14

By January of 1998, Carol, Elaine and I were trying to accept the fact that Carol would be unable to return to school. One of her greatest goals was to complete her education. Now it appeared that she would be unable to accomplish that goal.

Shortly after Carol entered the hospital for the last time, while she was still comatose, we received a call from Dr. Vance Davis, vice-president of High Point University. High Point's governing body had met and agreed that Carol's extracurricular activities was enough to grant her the last three semester hours of credit she needed to graduate. Carol would receive her diploma! I cried. I knew that Carol, if she knew, would be elated. I knelt beside her and whispered the news in her ear. I was so afraid that she didn't understand.

Several days later, Carol roused from her coma. At first, her mind was addled, and she couldn't comprehend much. As the days progressed, she grew more alert. I believe, before the end came, she did understand about her degree. I hope so. When we wrote her obituary, we proudly listed graduate of High Point University as one of her accomplishments.

I assumed that High Point would mail her diploma to us at semester's end. Instead, Dr. Davis wrote a letter inviting us to attend the graduation ceremony in May to receive Carol's diploma in her behalf. We were pleased to accept.

In the meantime, my work duties continued. The time for installation of our local area network (LAN) system approached. I was to be Hendersonville's Site LAN Coordinator. In SSA jargon, I was the "SLC" (pronounced slick). I was to attend a two week training session in Atlanta during early May. Coincidentally, the training schedule straddled the weekend of High Point's graduation. I made arrangements to leave Atlanta on Friday afternoon and return to Hendersonville. Elaine and I planned to travel to Winston-Salem on Friday night. Then we would make the half-hour trip to High Point Saturday morning for the graduation ceremony.

The first week of May, I traveled to Atlanta. Computers have always fascinated me. I am a charter member of the Hendersonville Area Computer Society, and I had the privilege of serving as president of the club for two years. As computer technology has progressed, however, I have been unable to stay current. Nonetheless, I understood much of what the instructors taught us that first week, so I felt good about that part of my responsibilities. I could see real possibilities for using this new system to improve the efficiency of our office. Perhaps the shock of Carol's death was wearing off.

I'm also a baseball fan. While I was in Atlanta, the Dodgers came to town, and I decided to visit Atlanta's new baseball stadium and take in a game. My hotel was on the outskirts of the city, right on I-285, the "belt" which encircled Atlanta. I hopped in my pickup and left for the game about two hours before time for the first pitch. I'll never do that again. When the first inning started, I was gridlocked in traffic, within sight of the stadium. I didn't get inside until the second inning was well underway. Next time, I'll take the MARTA public transit system. Once there, I found the game relaxing, anyway.

When class dismissed on Friday afternoon, I loaded my luggage (along with a week's worth of dirty clothes for washing at home), and headed north on I-85. I called Elaine to let her know about what time I would arrive. She was ready, and we loaded our 1997 GMC Jimmy and drove to Winston-Salem.

The thought of attending our daughter's posthumous graduation was another grim reminder of her absence. The three-hour trip was silent, as we pondered our memories of Carol. We made a point to arrive early Saturday morning, so we could get a decent parking place. We thought of the hectic hours the High Point students would spend packing for departure to their various homes. We also wanted some time to wander around campus and remember our times there with Carol. We went to the Annex, the small dorm where Carol had stayed. We peeked into the room that Carol had lived in, now occupied by another student. We remembered putting Carol's bed up on blocks so she could store more clothes under her bed. We remembered the day we brought Carol to interview for High Point's Presidential Scholarship program. That was on a Saturday in February of her senior year. Ice was on the parking lot, and Carol slipped and fell, splitting a seam in her new dress. Elaine was prepared, having stashed a sewing kit in her purse. She and Carol retreated to a restroom, where Elaine repaired the dress. High Point eventually awarded a full scholarship to Carol. We trudged across the way to the student center, where the High Point students had held a prayer vigil when Carol was so ill. We walked through the cafeteria, where Carol had eaten her meals.

Finally, we went to the large open area in front of Roberts Hall, where the graduation ceremonies were to be held. The custodial staff had placed hundreds of chairs in front of a large stage. The students would sit in the chairs to the left, the parents and friends would sit to the right. We met with Dr. Davis, who asked us to sit on the front row on the right side. He explained that we would be given Carol's diploma after the speeches and after the presentation of the diploma to the class president – before the rest of the diplomas were given out.

I was numb again, overwhelmed by grief over the loss of my daughter. I know Elaine felt the same way. The dignitaries were introduced, and the speeches were given. The sense of unreality I felt was palpable. Finally, Dr. Jacob Martinson announced the presentation of Carol's diploma, Magna Cum Laude. I wept uncontrollably as Elaine and I walked up the steps to the stage. as Dr. Martinson handed us the diploma, the entire student body rose and gave her a standing ovation. "Oh, look at that!" Dr. Martinson exclaimed. My tears blinded me so, I could hardly see.

After the ceremony, many of the professors and students came by to offer words of comfort and condolence to us. Many spoke fondly of the time they had spent with Carol, and how she had touched their lives. To this day, I treasure their words in my heart.

Later, Elaine and I returned to our car and got the small container which held a portion of Carol's ashes. We walked back to the Annex and scattered them around the perimeter of the building, saying a small prayer of thanksgiving for the good times Carol had enjoyed there. When Carol had first considered High Point as a possible location for her studies, I felt unsure about why she would be attracted to such a school. It was not as well known as some other schools on her list. In retrospect, I realize that she knew what she was doing. High Point is filled with loving, compassionate people who supported and encouraged her. No doubt this was the school God chose for her.

The following week, I returned to Atlanta to finish my "SLC" training. Because of my low energy reserves, two weeks of comprehensive training and a 700 mile round-trip to High Point and back left me exhausted. I returned to work worn out and still unable to make much of a substantial contribution.

The end of the school year at West Henderson High School approached. When Carol was at Rugby Junior High School, Glenda Lancaster was a guidance counselor there. She provided support when Carol and one of her school mates founded Rugby Against Alcohol and Drugs (RAAD) under the auspices of America's Pride, a national anti-drug organization. By 1998, America's Pride had a presence in most of the county junior and senior high schools. Glenda consulted Elaine and me about how the organization could honor Carol's memory. We suggested that the organization present a Carol Hooker Memorial award to the student who best demonstrated the principles of the Pride organization. Glenda liked the idea. When Honors Day came around at West, I had the privilege of presenting the award to the recipient.

The National Honor Society Chapter at West also decided to honor Carol by founding a scholarship in her name. During the same awards ceremony, I also helped present this award.

After Elaine completed her teaching duties for the semester, she and I went to Myrtle Beach, South Carolina. We needed a vacation, but we weren't up to a big one, and certainly not an expensive one. We visited a few sights, and spent the late afternoons walking along the beach in front of our hotel. When we lived in Petal, Mississippi, we often traveled to Navarre Beach, Florida during spring break. Carol was small then, and we enjoyed walking along the beach. We have a picture of Carol marching along the sands of Navarre Beach singing a song, in a world of her own. In 1997, at Carol's suggestion, we returned to Petal to visit friends and made one last trip (although we didn't know it at the time) to Navarre Beach.

During our walks along Myrtle Beach, Elaine and I solemnly recalled the fond moments we had spent with Carol at Navarre. It was a sad time, but a healing time. Gradually, my memories of the good times I had spent with Carol crept from the mental closet where they hid and pushed away some of the gruesome memories of Carol's illness and death.

Father's day arrived. I decided to send a card to my father, and to write in it a heartfelt thanks for all he had done for me. This is something I would never have been able to tell him personally, at least not without breaking down completely. In the card, I thanked him for teaching me about Christ, and for teaching me the many traits that I now consider so important. Those traits are honesty, integrity, responsibility and perseverance. Later, Mother told me how much that card meant to him.

Singer/songwriter Dan Fogelberg wrote a song of tribute for his father entitled, "Leader of the Band." There is a line in the song that says, "My life has been a poor attempt to imitate the man." That is how I feel. If I can live a life like my father's, I will be pleased, and I think God will be, too.

Dad was not a vocal person. He didn't have a lot of words to say. But his actions spoke volumes. I learned these things from him by example. Let me illustrate by telling about one event in my life.

When I was fifteen years old, and a student at Thaxton High School, I learned that the county school system had a program which hired some high school students to perform maintenance during the summer. I decided to apply. When I got to the county superintendents office, I learned that those hired had to be sixteen years old. So, I lied about my age, and I got hired. I believe I was to be paid the princely sum of $1.25 an hour. For a boy who usually spent his summers hoeing cotton for fifty cents an hour, this was good money.

I excitedly told my parents about my good fortune when I got home. I don't remember how they found out that I had lied to get hired, but they found out. Mom and Dad had to be tempted to let things ride, and to let me keep the job. Dad was somewhat miserly, and my earning some pocket money on my own would have eased my need for money from him. But he and Mother strongly believed in honesty.

Dad marched me back to the county school system office, where I had to confess and give up my job. I learned an important lesson. Money is less important than honesty. My parents taught me similar lessons about the other traits that have enabled me, as an adult, to respect myself and to respect others.

The next year, I got the job honestly. I spent the summer painting buildings and putting a new roof on the gymnasium.

I have spent some time researching the genealogy of my parents. I have been able to see that the things my father taught me are the same things his father taught him, and that his father taught him. The same thing applies on my Mother's side of the family.

As Carol grew into adulthood, Elaine and I were gratified to see her demonstrate those same traits. She was a Christian. She valued honesty, integrity and responsibility. She respected herself, and she respected others. I think one of the things that brought me the most pain was the realization that she would be unable to pass those gifts on to a child of her own.

We made plans to visit Mississippi during the week of July 4th. I was sure this would be the last time I would see my father alive. I was at work on June 30th, when I received a call from Mother telling me that I should come

49

immediately. She didn't think Dad would last much longer. Elaine and I packed quickly and we started on the ten hour journey to Mississippi. When we got to Chattanooga, about halfway, I called on our cell phone to see how Dad was doing. He had passed away about two hours before. Mom told me his death was very peaceful.

I regretted not being able to be there to say goodbye in person. I don't see how I could have made it, however. Since we didn't know his time was so near, I couldn't leave work and stay at his side forever. I know he knew what was in my heart, and we were able to say goodbye in spirit, if not in person.

So, I had to help plan a second funeral in six months. Browning Funeral Home in Pontotoc did the services. they did their usual fine job. Mom, my sister Pam and I selected a casket and arranged for the ceremony. We were undecided about whether to drape his casket with a flag, which he was due as a veteran, or with a spray of flowers. In the end, we decided to display the flag in a triangular display case beside the casket. That worked very well.

Our friends in and around Thaxton took good care of Mom and the rest of us, as I knew they would. Mom handled things very well. In his last days, Dad was serene in his fate. He knew he was going to Heaven. He had lived a long and fruitful life. That helped him achieve that serenity, and his serenity helped Mom, I believe. Personally, I was unsure about how I felt or was supposed to feel. My grief was not as deep as I had expected it to be. Perhaps it was because I was still struggling with my grief over Carol's death. Perhaps it was because Dad had lived a full life, and while none of us wanted him to die, it is something that happens to us all. So, Dad's death was more "normal" than Carol's had been. Nonetheless, I felt some guilt that I didn't feel emotions more strongly. All I could do about this ambivalence was to set it aside to deal with later.

William Carey is known as the father of missions. While in India, his five year-old son died and his wife went insane. During this crisis, he wrote, "This is indeed the valley of the shadow of death to me, except my soul is much more insensitive than John Bunyan's pilgrim...But I rejoice that I am here, not withstanding; and God is here, who not only can have compassion, but is able to save to the utmost."

CHAPTER SIX

My soul is in anguish. How long, O Lord, how long?
Psalm 6:3

"There is no way to resign from this…Suicide is out and I am afraid whatever I might try wouldn't work and I'd be back with this dreary ironing again. God is alive and working, but I feel as if I am in this tight box with the lid coming down, and no one can get to me."

Barbara Johnson;
Where Does A Mother Go to Resign?

In the months after Carol's death, I went through a distressing series of changes in behavior and attitude.

First I experienced a change in my sleep patterns, which began while I was in shock after my daughter died. Usually, I go to bed between 11:00 PM and midnight. After lying down, I now found myself unable to sleep. I tossed and turned, and lay awake for hours at a time. Often, I got up and went back to my living room to read. I sat there until 2:00, 3:00 or 4:00 AM. The next day I was groggy and less alert than I should have been, making it more difficult for me to do my job.

Conversely, I slept all day on Saturday and all afternoon on Sunday. On those days, I couldn't make myself do anything productive at all. I got up on Saturday morning, read the newspaper and ate breakfast, then piled onto the couch and slept until lunchtime. After lunch, I went back to the couch and slept until dinnertime. On Sunday, I went to church and Sunday School, ate lunch, then hit the couch for the afternoon. I know Elaine was worried about me, but there was little she could do.

Secondly, I was irritated and angry all of the time. I have claimed that I was not angry at God. I am still convinced that this is true. While I don't understand why Carol had to die at such an early age, I don't blame God for that. I had what psychologists call "unspecified anger". That is, I was angry at everything, and at nothing. I was just angry. If a leaf blew in front of my face, I was angry at the leaf. I knew my emotions were unfounded, and I struggled to keep them hidden, but it was a struggle. I didn't always succeed. I don't remember the incident, but Elaine tells of the time we went shopping at Lowe's Building Supply, and I nearly bit the head off a salesperson there for no good reason.

I do remember when Elaine and I went to the Asheville mall one Saturday (a rare one when I didn't sleep all day). While there, we decided to get cinnamon buns at one of the shops there. Cinnamon is one of my favorite spices. I ordered a large bun for me and a small one for Elaine. There was one small cinnamon bun left, but the clerk explained to me that the large ones were in the oven and I would have to wait only a few minutes for them to be ready. Okay, I said, I'll wait. While I waited, the clerk sold the last remaining small bun to another customer. Then the large ones came out of the oven. Now there were large buns, but no small ones! I lost my temper and berated the clerk for selling the last small bun, when I had already told her I wanted it. Clearly, the sales clerk didn't act appropriately, but I could have handled the situation more tactfully.

My third symptom was difficulty in making even the simplest decisions. This was most harmful to my work situation, since my job is to make decisions. I found myself struggling with problems that I couldn't find resolution for. The others in the office helped by keeping as much of the burden off me as possible, but it was still difficult. Each day was a struggle.

Lastly, I was laden with despair. Perhaps because I was unable to resolve problems, I couldn't find resolution for the symptoms I experienced. I only sank deeper into the morass. I could see no way out. Some people in this situation consider suicide. I did not, thanks to my reliance on God. I knew suicide was not an option. Nevertheless, I was mired in a pit of despair and I didn't know what to do. For a period of time in July, I contemplated resigning my position as manager of the Social Security office, and returning to the position of claims representative. The job of claims representative certainly isn't any easier than that of manager, but the scope of responsibility is less. I almost convinced myself that making that change would relieve me of some of the despair and helplessness that I felt.

I had read a lot about the grief process, and I knew that things usually got better over time. I tried to hang on and allow time to pass in the hopes that I would feel better. By the end of July, I realized this wasn't happening. Stepping down as manager was such a final act. I also had the good sense to know that I was in no condition to make such a monumental decision. I needed to be in better control of my faculties.

I finally decided to see a therapist. I hoped that he would walk me through a few steps in helping me sort out my life, and help with a few of these big decisions that were hanging over me. I made an appointment with Eli Machen, a Christian counselor who had an arrangement with First Baptist Church to counsel its members. I believed choosing a counselor with a Christian background to be wise. I have heard of non-Christian counselors whose advice involves having the patient put himself ahead of God, his family, and everything else. A relative who underwent counseling was told not to worry about her husband. If she wanted to leave her husband, go ahead. Whatever she believed was best, that was the thing to do.

I wasn't prepared to place God or Elaine or anyone else in jeopardy emotionally or spiritually because of my problems. I wanted a counselor who would use Bible-based principles to advise me. So, Eli Machen was my choice.

It took Eli about thirty seconds to diagnose my condition as clinical depression. Of course! I had read about that in the grief books. I was in such bad shape, I was unable to recognize the condition in myself.

We talked at length about my grief. He remembered meeting Carol when we attended group sessions for cancer victims. He commented on his fond memories of her, which made me feel better. He asked, "How do you feel about Carol's death?"

"I know Carol is in Heaven," I answered. "And I know that she is better off there. My head says that I should be happy for that. But my heart ..."

"Your heart says you miss her, and you wish she were still here with you." He finished.

"Yes, that's exactly right."

"Don't deny your grief." Eli advised. "It is difficult for a Christian to begrudge a loved ones place in Heaven. Don't feel that way. It is natural to miss her, and to wish she were here. In order to continue through the grief process, you have to acknowledge your loss and acknowledge the pain that comes with it. That doesn't take anything away from God or Carol's place in Heaven."

We also talked about the change in my role as a parent. For the past twenty-one years, being a parent had been a big part of my life. Now, suddenly, that role had been taken away from me. Eli told me that I should be aware of that, and perhaps find another role to take its place. He assured me that nothing would ever take my daughters place (something I already knew), and that the new role I selected would not replace my prior role as father. Instead, it would provide a new avenue for God to use me in His work. That made sense. I told him about my efforts to write a book about Carol's life, and my desire to write for publication. Eli thought that was an excellent idea. I've met many people who have lost loved ones, and who have undertaken creative endeavors as a means of therapy for their grief. I have met those who have written in journals, or who have written poetry, or who have written poems, and all of those efforts have proven beneficial.

At the end of my session, he recommended that I make an appointment with my family doctor to get an anti-depressant prescription. Overall, I saw Eli four times. During those sessions, we talked about working through the grief process.

Clinical depression is a medical condition, just like diabetes or any other illness. In diabetes, the body fails to produce the proper amount of insulin, and the body's systems don't function properly. In clinical depression, the brain fails to produce the proper amount of two chemicals called neurotransmitters: norepinephrine and serotonin. When these two chemicals are not in the right balance, the body's systems function improperly. Sleep patterns are disrupted. The victim is unable to think clearly, and unable to make even simple decisions. Irrational emotions run rampant. In some cases, the victim considers suicide.

William Styron, author of such best-selling novels as *The Confessions of Nat Turner* and *Sophie's Choice,* is one of many depression sufferers. Styron chronicled his illness in his book, *Darkness Visible*, and described his suicidal thoughts as follows. "He (a psychiatrist) asked me if I was suicidal, and I reluctantly told him yes. I did not particularize – since there seemed no need to – did not tell him that in truth many of the artifacts of my house had become potential devises for my own destruction: the attic rafters (and an outside maple or two) a means to hang myself, the garage a place to inhale carbon monoxide, the bathtub a vessel to receive the flow from my opened arteries. The kitchen knives in their drawers had but one purpose for me."

In my case, thoughts of suicide did not come into play. I am not sure why. Perhaps it was the realization that I could not leave Elaine with another death to deal with, or perhaps my heavy reliance on God shielded me from that option. I knew that suicide would serve no purpose in God's plan. In any case, I had to see this through, and that thought gave me the impetus to find help.

No one is immune from depression. It strikes rich and poor, white and black (and yellow and red). It strikes people of all religions and nationalities. It seems to strike more women than men, although I am not sure why, unless it is because women are more in touch with their emotions and thus more susceptible to the ravages of the disease.

Many people of note have suffered from the disease, and many of those have shared their experiences. Kathy Cronkite wrote a book about depression entitled *On the Edge of Darkness*. In it, she quotes some of these. Mike Wallace, CBS News anchorman said, "I didn't know what was the matter with me. All I knew was that I was feeling lower than a snake's belly…I remember we used to go to restaurants, and I'd say 'Everybody's pointing at me, the cheat, the fraud, the fake.' You really believe these things! Astonishing"

Rod Steiger said, "When you're depressed, there's no calendar. There are no dates, there's no day, there's no night, there's no seconds, there's no minutes, there's nothing. You're just existing in this cold, murky, ever-heavy atmosphere, like they put you inside a vial of mercury."

Once again, from William Styron's *Darkness Visible:* "It was not really alarming at first, since the change was subtle, but I did notice that my surroundings took on a different tone at certain times: the shadows of nightfall seemed more somber, my mornings were less buoyant, walks in the woods became less zestful, and there was a moment during my working hours in the late afternoon, when a kind of panic and anxiety overtook me."

Nathaniel Hawthorne wrote, "I have secluded myself from society; and yet I never meant any such thing. I have made a captive of myself and put me into a dungeon, and now I cannot find the key to let myself out."

Abraham Lincoln wrote, "I am now the most miserable man living. If what I feel were equally distributed to the whole human family, there would be not one cheerful face on earth. Whether I shall ever be better, I cannot tell. I awfully forbode I shall not. To remain as I am is impossible. I must die or be better it appears to me."

Winston Churchill suffered from frequent episodes of depression that he called, "The Black Dog."

All this because two little chemicals aren't produced in the proper proportions! Fortunately, there are medicines available today which offer help. I made an appointment with Dr. Tom Lugus, my family doctor. I described my conversation with Eli, and my symptoms. He immediately agreed with the diagnosis. He prescribed a medication called Paxil. He warned me that the medicine required a while to take effect. He said it might take up to a month to notice any difference in my symptoms. It may have taken a month for me to feel the full effects of the medication, but within a week I could tell a difference.

The utter despair I felt began to lift, ever so slightly at first, but even that little change was like breathing that first breath of fresh air in the spring. Over the next few weeks, my attitude improved. I still carried a lot of the grief that had burdened me so. And I still had the complex requirements of my work, so life didn't suddenly become wonderful. But I did feel at least, that I could get up each morning and show up for life.

Please allow me a moment to comment on how a friend or family member can help a victim of depression. To an onlooker, even one who cares, the depression victim may seem to be lazy, or even lolling in a "pity-party". Please remember that your loved one is unable to help himself in this condition. Admonishing him or her to "snap out of it" may only add guilt to the emotions they deal with. Many times I knew I had responsibilities I needed to fulfill, but I was unable to do anything. As an interested on-looker, the best help you may be able to offer is to guide the victim to get professional help. Perhaps even to help them see their condition.

I wasn't aware that I was suffering from clinical depression until Eli Machen pointed it out to me. Once he did, I was surprised that I hadn't realized it myself. The disease often masks itself from the victim. Some time after my own diagnosis, I noticed these same symptoms in a friend. I sat down with this friend, and described my condition, the symptoms I had experienced and compared them to the behavior my friend was exhibiting. Perhaps God allowed me to suffer this illness so I could be more compassionate toward others who had the same problem.

I think this was the low point in my grief. I had many more months to go before my journey would end – as I write this it has been three years since Carol's death, and I still do not believe my journey is over, perhaps it never will be – but I have never felt as hopeless as I did at this time in my life.

Here are some of the symptoms which may indicate the presence of clinical depression:

♦ A sad, anxious or empty mood which lasts for two or more weeks.

- A loss of interest or pleasure in most activities you once enjoyed.
- Feelings of worthlessness, hopelessness or guilt.
- Significant changes in sleep habits, which may include sleeping too much or too little.
- Fatigue or loss of energy.
- Agitation, restlessness or irritability.
- Difficulty in concentrating or making decisions.
- Frequent thoughts of death or suicide.

If you or someone you know is having these symptoms, you or she should see a doctor immediately. Clinical depression may be caused by the onset of another illness or injury which upsets the body's chemistry. It may also result from heredity, postpartum changes, medications or drug or alcohol abuse. One in five (20%) of Americans will be affected by depression in their lifetime, so while you may feel that you are alone in this malady, you are not. In most cases, medication can help. (This information came from a booklet entitled, "Depression: Getting the Help You Need," published by SmithKline Pharmaceuticals © 1997).

When I read the Psalms, I am convinced that David suffered from depression. He often lamented the seeming hopelessness of his situation. His answer was to call out to God for help and understanding. Once again, we can learn from this man of God. I believe that prayer is an important therapy for the treatment of depression. God is strong enough to carry our woes. He loves us and hears our prayers.

The question arises; why not just rely on God to lift our depression and not worry about taking medication or seeing a doctor? Don't forget that God is the Creator of all things. He is the source of healing that doctors and medicines provide. In short, seeing a doctor and taking medication is how God heals us – at least one of the ways. I am not going to be so presumptuous as to turn my back on the medical profession and foreclose that opportunity for God to provide healing.

In my case, that is exactly the means that God chose to provide relief for my depression.

CHAPTER SEVEN

The Lord is my rock, my fortress and my deliverer.
My God is my rock, in whom I take refuge.
He is my shield and the horn of my salvation, my
stronghold.

Psalm 18:2

About the time I started on the anti-depressant medication, things got really wild at the office. Until now, we used "dumb terminals" to connect to a small mini-computer in our data communications room, which in turn was connected by phone line to our mainframe computers in Baltimore. This allowed us to record the information necessary to take and process claims, and to input post-entitlement actions such as changes of address. These dumb terminals didn't allow us to prepare notices, or to record most of our administrative data. To do this we had to go to one of two "stand-alone" computers. With 16 people, we often had to wait in line for a chance to do our work. Additionally, our only means of electronic mail – email – was on one of the stand-alones. Our only email communication was with other Social Security offices.

The installation of a LAN system allowed us to put "smart" Pentium computers on each employee's desk. These computers were connected on a "ring" to a master server in the data communications room, which in turn was connected to the mainframes in Baltimore. This system allowed us to compose and print notices from our desks and to use many other programs not previously available to us. In addition, each of us had our own email capability. Our administrative functions were also on-line, which would make my job easier – once it was installed.

On Thursday, a delivery truck trundled up to our building and disgorged box after box of computer hardware. A systems engineer from Unisys arrived shortly thereafter. That night, he installed the server, which housed most of the software the employees would use. Each employee's computer accessed the software from the server, and saved computer disk space.

When we closed for business on Friday night, the engineer and a team of assistants installed the new computers on the desks of each employee. I was on hand to assist, along with Terry Parker and Vanessa White, the systems coordinator from Asheville. When the engineering team completed the installation of a terminal, Terry, Vanessa or I would log onto the computer and work through a detailed checklist, testing each piece of hardware and software. We toiled until midnight. The anti-depressant had not yet begun its work. In fact, the first couple of doses made me even more of a zombie than usual. I felt disembodied, as if I was having an out-of-body experience. I watched myself from across the room as I completed the tests on each of the computers. If we'd had a serious problem, I'd have had to rely on Terry or Vanessa to resolve it. Fortunately, things went smoothly. Shortly after midnight, we signed off on the last computer and went home.

The following Monday, I felt more normal, although I still hadn't benefited much from the anti-depressant. We were in for a hectic week. The office staff had to undergo a week of indoctrination on the new system. We divided the staff into three teams. One team trained, a second team practiced the techniques they had just learned, working through exercises and experimenting a little as they went. The third team answered the phones and handled the daily workload, since we had to be open to the public as usual. After about half a day, the teams switched roles.

Several other Social Security offices were undergoing the same training we were. One of the tricky aspects was learning the intricacies of the email system. I received a "practice" email from an employee in a Virginia office. She thought she was sending it to a friend, when in fact, she sent it to all 65,000 Social Security employees! We were careful, and avoided that embarrassment.

At the end of the week, our training was completed. While I knew this new system would make us much more efficient. I feared that an employee or two might find themselves overwhelmed by the new system. Fortunately, everybody embraced the system joyfully. We still had a steep learning curve to go through, but everyone was on board and ready to maximize this new tool. I was lucky in another aspect, as well. Almost always, a new system has a few bugs buried in it, which cause problems. Our system worked almost perfectly. God was looking out for me in this fashion, as well.

Back in January, in the last few weeks before Carol's death, I resolved to try to write a book about her life. I had shared that goal with Eli, who encouraged me. He knew it would be good therapy for me, allowing me to work through the grief process. While writing the book, was difficult, it was indeed good therapy.

I tried to write for an hour or two every day. I spent hours going through old photo albums and old records, recalling special moments in my life with Carol. These mementos helped me recollect events that I used to chronicle her life. I went through the many cards that Carol had received, and those that Elaine and I had received after her death. I recorded excerpts from many of the notes that were included. I contacted Carol's friends and asked them to contribute some special memory they had. I also asked some of the people who sat with Carol during her last stay in the hospital to record something of that experience. Slowly the book came together.

After many months, the old closet that hid those positive memories of my daughter opened, and I was able to once again cherish the many good times she and Elaine and I had shared. That terrible mental picture of Carol's breathless body on the hospital bed appeared less often. The book was doing its job. Slowly, God provided healing.

I had another trial to endure, however. It was time to observe the first anniversaries of events in Carol's illness. I often found myself thinking, "On this day, last year, Carol had her first gastro-intestinal bypass surgery." On September 12, I remembered, "This is the day, Carol's cancer was diagnosed." These thoughts brought new remorse. Fortunately, the anti-depressant medication had taken effect, and these thoughts were not as overwhelming as they could have been. I knew the next few months would be arduous as I endured the recollections of Carol's last months, and the first holidays without her.

Thanksgiving has always been a low-key holiday for us. We never went in for a big dinner or parties. We also weren't big turkey fans. We usually bought a ham, which Elaine served with vegetables. This Thanksgiving was pretty much the same. Only without Carol, it was different, too. The house was altogether too silent. We had little joy. We didn't really feel thankful, although we knew we still had much to thank God for. I know He understood our feelings.

At Christmas, we made our usual trip to Mississippi. Elaine and I didn't feel like doing much Christmas shopping, so we arranged with family members to forego the exchange of gifts. While packing our car for the trip, Elaine marveled at our trip the previous Christmas. We have a 1997 GMC Jimmy – a mid-sized SUV. Last year, we not only packed our clothes and Christmas gifts, we also packed Carol's gastric suction machine and her enterol pump. Looking at the cargo compartment of the Jimmy, Elaine could not understand how we got everything packed. We decided that God stretch the Jimmy just a little bit last year to allow everything to fit.

We didn't know it at the time, but this trip would be the last Christmas we would spend with Papaw Pannell. Before the next Christmas rolled around, he would join his wife in Heaven. As it was, we could tell he was getting very feeble. His strength had diminished considerably, and he suffered from some confusion.

Shortly after we arrived, winter embraced us in her frigid arms. An ice storm moved in, and knocked Papaw's power out. Not only were we depressed from trying to celebrate Christmas without Carol, we were cold, as well.

In years past, we put the gifts under the tree after Carol went to bed on Christmas Eve. When we arose Christmas morning, we gathered around the tree to open gifts and admire each other's treasure. We still put the gifts under the tree on Christmas Eve, and still opened them the next morning, but with Carol absent we had little excitement to share and little interest in treasure. We just went through the motions.

Traditionally, Elaine's family gathered at Papaw's house for Christmas lunch, and opened gifts that afternoon. With the power out, we moved the celebration to Robert and Mary Ann Wigington's house. They lived on the other side of Ellistown and had been spared in the power outage.

I came from a small family, and our gatherings were always quiet and sedate. When I first joined Elaine's family, I often suffered headaches (from the noise) after one of their get togethers. With about fifty people in the house, there was a constant babble, somewhat like a flock of hens cackling. In my early years, I would sit to one side and try to count the number of simultaneous conversations going on. Usually, I just gave up. As I became accustomed to the family, the headaches no longer came, and I felt more comfortable joining in the conversations. This year, however, I was again off to one side, in a morose funk. I had no inclination to join in the cacophony. I could only remind myself that my daughter was gone, and would never be able to join in celebrating Christmas with us again.

I should have reminded myself that, no doubt, Carol was celebrating Christmas that day. Only she was celebrating it with the "Birthday Boy" Himself. My intellect knew that Carol was much better off in Heaven, where she enjoyed the fruits of her salvation and witness. But my heart could never quite grasp that fact, and I often immersed myself in my own grief over her loss. Eli Machen would have told me that is natural, and is to be expected, especially during the holiday season. Counselors emphasize that holidays are often the toughest time of year for grievers. I can only imagine how deep my depression would have been without the anti-depressant medication.

I knew Elaine was no better off. During all this time that I was wallowing in my own grief, she was dealing with the same emotions. One of the problems with grieving parents after the loss of a child is that each person must grieve and thus is incapable of offering support or comfort to the other person. Each person thrashes in his own sea of emotions. Elaine and I recognized this, and we tried to support each other as best we could. We reminded ourselves that on our wedding day, we each said, "'Til death do us part." So we committed to each other that we wouldn't let our grief ruin our marriage. While we had some rough spots through the year, we knew we would stick together.

We had another stage of Christmas tradition to fulfill after the Pannell get-together. We made the forty-five minute drive to Thaxton to spend Christmas night with my

Tom Hooker

Mom, my sister and her family. At Mom's, we toiled under a double whammy. Not only was Carol gone for the first time, Dad was too. On several occasions, we had to comfort each other as someone cried. Once again, the mood was somber. At least Mom had electricity, and we didn't have to endure the cold.

The next day, we returned to Papaw's and the day after that, we made the return trip to North Carolina. That Christmas will not go down as one of our favorites.

MY FIRST CHRISTMAS IN HEAVEN

I see the countless Christmas trees
around the world below
With tiny lights, like Heaven's stars
reflecting on the snow

The sight is so spectacular,
please wipe away the tear
For I am spending Christmas with
Jesus Christ this year

I hear the many Christmas songs
that people hold so dear
But the sounds of music can't compare
with the Christmas choir up here.

I have no words to tell you,
the joy their voices bring,
For it is beyond description,
to hear the angels sing.

I know how much you miss me,
I see the pain inside your heart.
But I am not so far away,
We really aren't apart.

So be happy for me, dear ones,
You know I hold you dear.
And be glad I'm spending Christmas
with Jesus Christ this year.

I sent you each a special gift,
from my heavenly home above.
I sent you each a memory
of my undying love.

After all, love is the gift more precious
than pure gold.
It was always most important
in the stories Jesus told.

Please love and keep each other,
as my Father said to do.
For I can't count the blessing or love
He has for each of you.

So have a Merry Christmas and
wipe away that tear.
Remember, I am spending Christmas with
Jesus Christ this year

A 13-year-old boy who died of a brain tumor wrote this poem. He died on December 14, 1997. He gave this to his mom before he died. His name was Ben.

CHAPTER EIGHT

"Everything that has happened to me has made me the woman I am today. I like that person. I respect her. She's courageous and honest. Regrets? Life did to me what life does. It presents you with opportunities, and sometimes it pushes you down, but it makes you what you are."

Della Reese, Parade Magazine,
December 17, 2000.

By January 1999, Carol's book was nearing completion. Before Carol became ill, I had toyed with the idea of doing some creative writing. I had an idea for a novel using the *Star Trek: The Next Generation* characters. I even wrote a rough draft. I called it *The Cardassian Border Incident*. I have to admit, it was very poorly written. I set the book aside, hoping for some creative magic to help me polish it up. Now, I am afraid, the plot is dated and is of no use. Perhaps one day I can adapt the plot to another set of characters and do something with it.

Writing Carol's book provided a great deal of education and experience for me. I know God was with me, because it came together so well, despite a slump in my writing when my depression episode was at its worst. I discovered that putting words on paper (or in a computer) is only the beginning. Each page has to be edited and re-written, and edited again. I made at least four editing passes on each chapter, sometimes more. I found repetitive phrases, redundant passages, passive sentences, and so on. I found that the real craft of writing is in the editing. I have done additional study on the subject, and have found that most writers have reached that same conclusion.

Now, with the book almost completed, I had to decide what to do with it. I had always intended to offer it to the public if I succeeded in completing it. But I wasn't sure if I could find a publisher, To sell a book like this one, the subject of the book almost has to be a celebrity. While Carol had definitely made an impact on the lives of many people in Hendersonville and High Point, I didn't believe she was well known enough for a "name" publisher to accept it. I also knew that the publishing process pursued by established publishing houses would mean a wait of eighteen to twenty-four months before the book would be available to the public. I wasn't prepared to wait that long.

That left the option of self-publishing. I'd have to finance the book myself, as well as handle the production, marketing and distribution. I decided that was what God would have me do. I didn't expect to profit from the book, that was not what my effort was all about. I decided breaking even was an appropriate goal. I am happy to say that, with God's help, I met that goal.

I needed a title. My first choice was *In His Grip*. That was the way Carol always closed her letters, and I thought it aptly described what her life was all about. My research revealed that another book had already been published using that title. While copyright laws to not apply to titles, and I could have legitimately used it, I feared that some confusion might arise as a result. Another title came to mind, put there, no doubt, by God. That title was *Calvary's Child*. That title also described Carol. I added *The Life of Amanda Carol Hooker* as a subtitle.

Publishing a book is like producing a movie. The publisher is responsible for all aspects of making the book come to life. Many well-known authors have used self-publishing as a means of marketing their work at one time or another. Pat Conroy, the author of such best-sellers as *Beach Music, The Prince of Tides, The Lords of Discipline, and The Great Santini*, tells an amusing story about his experiences with self-publishing. When Conroy wrote his first book, he was unfamiliar with the business of publishing. With the advice of a lawyer friend, he anted up the money to self-publish it. Later, after he had written his second novel, his lawyer friend decided to offer it to a publishing house, which offered an advance of $5000 for it. The lawyer called Conroy and told him, "They said they would do it for $5000.00."

Conroy was dismayed. "I don't have that much money." He said. Now, of course, his advances are substantially more than that.

After some research, I decided to hire Morris Publishing Company in Nebraska to print the book for me. They offered a good instructional package which helped me to select a suitable cover layout, and to make reasonably good decisions about formatting, fonts etc. I was getting a real education in the business of book publishing. I learned that by submitting the book in "camera-ready" format, I could avoid paying typesetting costs. While it was tedious, the effort was worth it.

I wanted to do things right. I knew I needed to follow the parameters of the law. I set up a sole proprietorship company, named Stoney Mountain Press, and registered it at the county Register of Deeds office. I established a business account. I obtained an employer identification number from the IRS, and recorded the company with the State Department of Revenue. I obtained as ISBN number for the book, and registered it with the U.S. Copyright office and with the Library of Congress. Whew!

Next, I had to make decisions about marketing the book. About the time I sent the manuscript off to the printer, I prepared a direct mail campaign to those who had sent cards to Carol or to Elaine and me. I also sent a mailing to the members of our church in Hendersonville, and my old church in Thaxton. In short, anyone I thought might be interested in reading the book got a letter from Stoney Mountain Press.

The response was gratifying. By the time the completed book was back from Morris Publishing, I had sold almost all of my initial order. I immediately ordered a second printing. I contacted the Hendersonville *Times-News*, our local newspaper, and they were kind enough to do an article, as did the student newspaper at High Point University.

Things were going well, but I still had a lot to learn about marketing. I blithely assumed that bookstores would fall all over themselves to stock the book on their shelves. I mailed a marketing kit to a number of bookstores in North Carolina and Mississippi. I received only one small order from a bookstore in Tupelo Mississippi. I made personal visits to stores in the Hendersonville area. I was sure that they would be excited about stocking the book, since Carol's home was here. I received a cool reception, however. While none of the bookstore owners or managers explained, I managed to learn about my *faux pas*. Independent bookstores do not purchase books directly from a publisher. Upon contemplation, that makes sense. There are hundreds of publishers, and bookstores – especially small ones – don't want to handle invoices from each individual publisher. Instead, they buy their books from a distributor, who buys the books from the publisher. That way, the bookstore owner only has to handle invoices from one or two distributors.

The largest book distributor in the country is Ingram's, located in La Vergne Tennessee. Of course, their primary interest is in larger publishers, and some little one-book publisher from Hendersonville North Carolina is outside their area of concern. I learned that Ingram's does have a program for small publishers who met a specific set of criteria. The publisher has to be a member of the Publishers Marketing Association, a national organization of small publishers who pool their resources to market their books. After joining PMA, I signed up for one of their promotional packages. I then submitted a report to Ingram's on what Stoney Mountain Press had to offer, and how I would handle promotion and marketing. God smiled again. Ingram's accepted Stoney Mountain Press into its program and listed *Calvary's Child* in its inventory.

Amazon.com is a large on-line bookstore which has pioneered Internet marketing. They also have a program for small publishers. I completed an application for their program, sent a copy of *Calvary's Child* for their review, and uploaded a computer image of the book cover. Amazon.com accepted my application. Now *Calvary's Child* is available through that website. Lastly, Barnes & Noble set up an account for me, and I have sold several books through that chain. Books-A-Million has also purchased a small number.

During this process, I learned a lot about the writing and publishing industry. I learned also that, despite my suffering, I was still able to see a project through to completion. God gave me the impetus to write and self-publish *Calvary's Child* to promote my own healing as well as to perpetuate Carol's witness. Once again, I learned how tragedy can be used for God's Glory.

As I had hoped, the book was well received. Here are a few of the comments that readers sent to me:

"I came home Saturday after the Mensa Executive Committee meeting and started reading *Calvary's Child* about 9:30, planning on reading about thirty minutes. Instead, I finished about 2:30 AM, dried my tears and went to bed.

"It's a lovely book – thank you for giving me a chance to meet Carol through its pages. What an extraordinary young woman you and Elaine raised – and how many other people have been reached, and their lives uplifted, because of this child you and Elaine nurtured and guided.

"Thank you for your honesty about mulligans – all of us who have been caretakers have a few of those. Even when you know you did the best your energy would permit, you wish somehow you'd managed to meet every need – and felt the humbling of accepting that our human selves can never meet all the needs of another." Mary Fond Daughtridge, Brevard NC.

"I've really been enjoying the book. Speaking for myself, I find the reading just compelling – 'once you start, you just can't put it down.' kind of experience. And, I've also got to tell you I was so impressed and praise God for the way Carol's influence and witness affected so many people – especially the professors at High Point who came to know the Lord through Carol's witness. I truly think Carol's life through *Calvary's Child* will continue to influence people for God's Kingdom. Let me say, too, that I personally enjoyed the information on your and Elaine's early time together before and after you were married. Tom, I also can and still do, identify with your struggles as a father as you so honestly related and Elaine, I'm sure when Pam reads the book, she will certainly be able to empathize with your experience as a mother.

"Finally, let me say how I admire Carol for her persistence in being the person God wanted her to be in the face of all her health problems, and these were not just usual aches and pains. She was *so* faithful to the Lord. Would to God that I, ... that we all could maintain the kind of witness Carol exhibited in this world of darkness. How her light did shine!

"So, until later, thanks for sharing – I know there has to be a bittersweet joy in knowing how the book is being received, but the consolation is still strong in that Carol is still being faithful to God through your thoroughly captivating account of her life." Joe Sewell, The Colony, TX.

"Tommy, I just wanted to let you know that I finished your book, and I believe the Lord inspired you in your writing. What a sweet, evangelistic message. What victory Carol had when she arrived at the feet of Jesus. Thank you so much for sharing your joy and your sorrow." James. A. & Diann Sullivan, Fort Lauderdale, FL.

"I wanted to read your book since I knew so little about Carol's illness and death, and though I did not contact you at the time, I was very concerned from the sketchy reports that I got. I did pray for you and your family. After reading the book I feel that I know you better, and my heart truly goes out to you and Elaine. From the little that you had told me about Carol, I knew that she was a special person and your book made me realize that anew. She was fortunate to have the two of you for parents.

"Two things came to mind after I finished reading. How did you keep up with the dates and what happened when? So much happened and the trips to doctors and hospitals must have run together in your mind. You did a great job of telling how and when things happened and the pinpointing of the actual drugs and tests was meaningful. The other thing is I am so thankful that you made a church connection in Hendersonville long before this illness befell Carol. So often people fail to do that, and then they are so alone when something happens and their families are two or three states away. I know you both would have welcomed having family close by, but the church obviously gave you lots of support when you needed it most.

"I have always said that there are things that we will have to ask St. Peter when we get to Heaven, and this is a classic question. Your summation that God has plans for your life and witness is an insightful conclusion. There are so many things that we cannot understand, and must accept on faith.

"Her accomplishments in her short life were truly impressive. Any college student who witnesses to a professor is unusual, and leading that person to make a profession of faith is almost unheard of. I certainly could not have done that at that stage in my own life, though I was a professing Christian." Mary Cain, Raleigh NC.

"I wanted to thank you for introducing me to Carol. I think I may have seen her a couple of times. I don't even know if we ever had a conversation. After reading *Calvary's Child* I feel that I know her well. She was truly a remarkable person. Her life has inspired me to walk even closer to our Lord. Her life on this earth may be over, but God is still using the life she lived to draw others closer to Him. I teach a youth group at our church. I have used a few passages from your book with them, such as the letter to her future husband, her letter to God, and some of her talks about drug abuse. I even had one of the girls ask to read the book. She has finished it and is encouraging others to read it also. I know God has blessed me through the life of Carol Hooker." Annalisa Hooker Spears, Thaxton, MS.

CHAPTER NINE

"Not only so, but we rejoice in our sufferings, because we know that suffering produces perseverance, perseverance produces character; and character, hope."

Romans 5:3-4

"Of course, life is possible without God. So many desperate people, they survive with nothing but themselves. But hope? Who can stand alone and still know this?"

T. Davis Bunn, *Drummer in the Dark*

It was now March 1999. Thirteen months since Carol died. Time to evaluate where I stood in my life. I am going to "think out loud", so these remarks may be a little disjointed.

I consider myself an optimist. My definition of an optimist is one who chooses to be happy, no matter what, whereas a pessimist is one who chooses to be unhappy, no matter what. Circumstances do not make optimists, attitudes do. Goodness knows, I have plenty of reasons to be unhappy. I know this book is filled with pain, but please remember, this is THE low point in my life. I knew that, while I would always miss Carol, I would go on with my life. It was up to me to choose how I would approach the rest of my life.

I know that one day, I will be in Heaven. I know that, one day, I will encounter the joy that Carol experiences right now. That is why I choose to look up instead of looking down. Some people believe that when we get to Heaven, we won't recognize those we knew here on earth. I believe that we will. I believe that Elaine and I will one day

79

be with Carol again. We may not be together as parent and child, instead we may be as children of God. But I believe we will be reunited.

I know that I am changed forever. While my grief will one day be less, I will carry a scar forever, and that scar will affect my life. I will always have an emotional limp. My job is to find a way to live for God's glory, even with that handicap.

I have come to realize that with love comes grief. Grief is the counterbalance to love. Very few people in a love relationship, whether it be as parent and child, or as husband and wife, or as friends, have both members of that relationship die simultaneously. When one member dies first, the other must grieve. Because we love, we grieve. The deeper our love for the person we have lost, the deeper our grief. Grief is not a bad thing, although it is painful. It is a means of disengaging from our loved one. It is a means of healing from our loss.

Losing a loved one is like losing a part of your body. Dr. Terese A. Rando, in her book *Grieving: How to Go On Living When Someone You Love Dies*, had this to say, "Your children, have sprung from you. They are a part of you and, consequently, in some ways are the same as you. In this way losing your child means losing parts of yourself. One bereaved mother described it this way, 'When you lose your spouse, it is like losing a limb; when you lose your child, it is like losing a lung.'"

Once, when Carol was ill, Bruce Ashe, a friend and fellow church member visited me at work. He commented that he didn't understand how Elaine and I endured the crisis of having a daughter at death's door. I told him that courage had nothing to do with it, we endured it because we had no choice. I think Bruce was expecting some noble response, and was surprised. In *A Grief Observed*, C.S. Lewis wrote, "Aren't all these notes the senseless writings of a man who won't accept the fact that there is nothing we can do with suffering except to suffer it?" Quite so.

On the other hand, God's presence is a help. I do believe that if God had not been at my side, I would have committed suicide, or attempted it. Why would continuing to live serve any purpose if there was nothing beyond life to look forward to? With God beside me, however, I know that this world is not the end. There is an eternal life beyond. I know that Carol is in Heaven. Even if we don't know each other when we reach The Golden City, that knowledge is enough to convince me that continuing to live for God and for my wife is worthwhile. So I continue.

First Baptist Church's Easter program in 1999 was entitled, "God for Us". Part of the program involved church members sharing about how God helped them through some crisis. Wally Shamburger, FBC's minister of music, asked me to share my experiences. Here is the text of my presentation:

"In Romans 8:28 we read, 'And we know that in all things God works for the good of those who love Him, who have been called according to His purpose.'

"Thirteen months ago, Carol Hooker, my 21 year old daughter, died after struggling with health problems for several years, including - ultimately - cancer.

"Carol accepted Christ at age 7, and grew to love her Savior dearly. This love inspired her to lean on God and to learn from God as she grew older. When her health problems began, she was prepared to use them as a ministry tool.

"During her years of illness, Carol used that illness to demonstrate how God offered strength in the midst of her trials; and she demonstrated that even illness was a means to glorify God.

"She shared that witness with many groups, inlcuding America's Pride, Fellowship of Christian Athletes, and Campus Crusade for Christ. She shared that witness with the youth of this church at Disciple Now and through other youth activities, and she shared that witness with children and adults in the Bahamas through Island Outreach.

"She shared God's love with her teachers at school and her professors at college, four of whom accepted Christ as their Savior, with her classmates and with the doctors, nurses and visitors in her hospital room. Those whose visits sought to lift her spirits found theirs lifted instead.

"During Carol's last year, she used a daily devotion book from the Experiencing God series. On October 26 — 6 weeks after she was diagnosed with cancer and three and 1/2 months before her death — she wrote these words in the margin:

"'Through the cancer God has brought revival to my heart again. Never before have I longed for Him as I do now to feel his presence and strength. Thank God for cancer.'

"In the weeks after Carol's death we received cards from Carols friends by the bucketsful. These friends shared how their lives had been changed by God's work in Carol's life. This outpouring of love helped us in our grief, but it also taught us that from our daughter's death a good thing happened. People grew closer to God.

"Romans 8:28 assures us that there is nothing — not one thing — that cannot be used to glorify God. It is a verse which promises that in everything bad, there is something good. In every tragedy, there is hope, in every tear, there is a blessing. This verse is also a reminder that hard things happen in every Christian life. But these hard things are opportunities. We must seek God's strength to harvest them. It is that assurance that gives my wife Elaine and me the strength to say, "Thank God for the grief of losing a child."

My Father's Hand

I sought a place
where pain was unknown.
I found a place
where comfort was sown.

I sought a place
where grief became unfounded
I found a place
where solace grew unbounded.

I sought a place
which soothed my fears
I found a place
which welcomed my tears.

The place I found
the place I stand
is in the palm of My Father's hand.

Tom Hooker

"The melody that the loved one played upon the piano of your life will never be played quite that way again, but we must not close the keyboard and allow the instrument to gather dust. We must seek out other artists of the spirit, new friends who gradually will help us find the road to life again, who will walk that road with us."

Joshua Liebman, *Peace of Mind*

Tom Hooker

EPILOGUE

"'Go at once to Zarepeth of Sidon and stay there. I have commanded a widow in that place to supply you with food.' So he went to Zarepath. When he came to the town gate, a widow was there gathering sticks. He called to her and asked, 'Would you bring me a little water in a jar so I may have a drink?' As she was going to get it, he called, 'And bring me, please, a piece of bread.'

"'As surely as the Lord your God lives,' she replied, 'I don't have any bread – only a handful of flour in a jar and a little oil in a jug. I am gathering a few sticks to take home and make a meal for myself and my son, that we may eat it – and die.'

"Elijah said to her, 'Don't be afraid. Go home and do as you have said. But first make a small cake of bread for me from what you have and bring it to me, and then make something for yourself and your son. For this is what the Lord, the God of Israel, says; "The jar of flour will not be used up and the jug of oil will not run dry until the day the Lord gives rain on the land."'

"She went away and did as Elijah had told her. So there was food every day for Elijah and for the woman and her family. For the jar of flour was not used up and the jug of oil did not run dry, in keeping with the word of the Lord spoken by Elijah."

I Kings 17:9-16

In mid-1998, I spent a lot of time considering the option of leaving my position as manager of the Hendersonville Social Security office and returning to the position of claims representative. I decided not to do that for several reasons. First, I knew that my grief had reached its lowest point (I hoped), and that my mind wasn't clear enough to make a major career decision like that. Second, I was concerned about the financial impact this change would have on Elaine and me. Making that change would reduce my income by about 25%. I didn't know if our budget could take such a hit. Third, I believed that making that change would be giving up. It would be admitting failure, and I didn't like that concept. I believed that going back to claims rep would mean that the grief had won. Perhaps, at that time, it would have been true.

By June 2001, I was still struggling with my situation at work. The demands of the job were placing such stress on me that I was concerned about my health. I had to accept the fact that I was burned out; assisted, no doubt by the drain on my energy that my grieving had caused. I reached the conclusion that if I were to consider my long-term health, I must reduce the stressors in my life. I still feared that this would represent a failure on my part. I was not accustomed to moving backward on the career ladder. I believed that I was clear-headed enough now to make a rational decision, but I still was unsure what this change would mean to our financial health. I made numerous financial projections, taking into account the reduced state and federal income tax deductions that my change in income would entail. I talked at length with Elaine, who shared my concerns. Elaine had gone through similar stresses at her workplace. I had hoped to put us in a position that would allow Elaine to resign from her job if or when she felt it necessary. I was aware that my career change would jeopardize that option for Elaine. Nevertheless, I didn't think I had a choice. Finally, I chose to request reassignment to claims rep effective July 1st.

By December 2001, six months later, I was able to assess the results of that change. Once again, the Lord has taken care of us. My stress level dwindled immediately. I threatened to make a sign to put on my desk which said "NMP". That meant "Not My Problem." No longer did I carry the responsibility of the entire office on my shoulders. I didn't have to worry about having enough people on hand to do the work. I didn't have to worry about union issues. I didn't have to worry about maintaining the equipment or the office space. It was "Not My Problem!" I was also pleasantly surprised at how much fun I was having as a claims representative. As manager, most of the members of the public that I spoke to were people who were having trouble with Social Security, or were angry with us about something. As a result, these people were usually angry or frustrated or scared. As a claims rep, I interviewed people who were first contacting us about filing for Social Security. Sometimes they were apprehensive, and I tried to put them at ease, but rarely were they already angry. I also had the opportunity to prevent the occurrence of problems which might send them to the manager in the future. I had forgotten how much fun it was to routinely "rub elbows" with members of the public. I could crack jokes and make their contact with Social Security fun and relatively stress-free. In short, it was fun. Anther aspect of the claims rep job involved taking claims from survivors of deceased workers – widows and children. I found that my experience with grief helped me to be more empathetic regarding their plight. Often, I just listened while they talked about their loss. At other times I offered encouragement. God had returned me to a place where I could use my experience with loss the ease someone else's burden.

God also took care of us financially. We hardly noticed the change in our income. Like the widow that Elijah instructed to dip flour from the empty bucket, we just didn't run out! I am always concerned when I relate a testimony like this that I may give someone the impression that God won't let financial hardship befall one of his children. I can't make that promise. I have seen Christian brothers and sisters encounter financial hardships, and I believe a crisis like that can apply to a Christian just as much as the crisis of losing a child. However, in this instance, things worked out for us financially, and I believe God had a hand in it.

I had one other issue to consider. Did moving back down the career ladder from manager to claims representative mean I had failed? Did the grief win? I suppose that depends on the criteria one uses to make that judgement. Someone who measures success by the amount of money a person makes or the amount of power a person wields might decide that I had failed. I am reminded that God uses a different yardstick to measure success or failure. I have always defined success as "living in God's will and achieving happiness" (which I think are synonymous). Using this measure, I don't think I failed. I still believe I am in God's will, and I am happier now than I was during my last several years as manager. So, I accept that the steps that I took were the right ones.

ABOUT THE AUTHOR

Tom Hooker was born and raised in the farm country of Pontotoc County Mississippi, about 100 miles southeast of Memphis, Tennessee. He received a business degree from the University of Mississippi in 1972, and has served as a claims representative, operations supervisor, branch manager and district manager with the Social Security Administration for the last twenty-five years. He is a member of the Hendersonville NC First Baptist Church, where he teaches Sunday school and is a deacon. He is a member of Mensa, and of the Hendersonville Area Computer Society. He donates platelets regularly with the American Red Cross. He and the former Elaine Pannell recently celebrated their thirtieth wedding anniversary.

Printed in the United States
4504

9 781403 302342